chronic disease nursing

a rheumatology example

Edited by **Susan M Oliver** RGN, MSc

Independent Rheumatology Nurse Specialist, North Devon

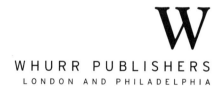

WHURR PUBLISHERS

LONDON AND PHILADELPHIA

© 2004 Whurr Publishers Ltd
First published 2004
by Whurr Publishers Ltd
19b Compton Terrace
London N1 2UN England and
325 Chestnut Street, Philadelphia PA 19106, USA

British Library Cataloguing in Publication Data

A catalogue record for this book
is available from the British Library.

ISBN 1 86156 412 0

Typeset by Adrian McLaughlin, a@microguides.net
Printed and bound in the UK by Athenæum Press Limited, Gateshead, Tyne & Wear

Contents

Preface

These are exciting yet challenging times for nurses. In the last few years the contribution of nurses and practitioners has been recognised and yet, along with this recognition comes the hope that we can develop appropriate services. For chronic disease patients the support of specialist expertise is imperative. Providing this support is no small task with the increasing elderly and chronic disease population and spiralling healthcare costs, accompanied by a shortage of healthcare professionals.

This book aims to provide practical support to the new or aspiring nurse in chronic disease care whether they work in primary or secondary care. Although the examples used in this book are those from the rheumatology community, they have relevance to other areas and can provide nurses with an insight into why nurses are recognised as key players in healthcare as well as how to make the best of this new found recognition.

From my own personal experience there seemed to be a dearth of books that provided a step wise approach to many new 'service development needs' or business planning proposals. Much of the information was learned by word of mouth, luck or trial and error! The jargon that managers used and the pitfalls in planning the appropriate resources for service delivery are all potential minefields for the enthusiastic but uninformed! Healthcare services can ill afford to lose valuable nurses who become disillusioned with trying to improve care and fall foul of inappropriate planning and unresourced services. It is for this reason that the first two chapters set the framework for the provision of specialist nursing care. Chapters one and two provide the background to the development of nursing and go on to explain how to identify the infrastructure and resources required to develop a service.

Telephones have become an essential component of everyday life and their use has been shown to provide a wealth of support to individuals in a range of settings with minimal overheads. Equally in the provision of chronic disease care they provide an essential and efficient method of supporting the patient at a time of uncertainty or need. Yet for many the telephone helpline services have been developed in an ad hoc way, with good intentions and often no funding. Telephone helpline services are not without risk. In fact it could be argued that providing safe and effective clinical support using only the telephone as a means of communication is fraught with potential problems. Chapter three provides the nurse with an understanding of some of the issues that need to be considered when setting up a helpline service.

Three chapters are structured around nurse led clinics. They include advice on the considerations that a nurse must make before setting up a clinic and why it is important to consider the use of various outcome measures. Although historically nurses have been recognised for their valuable contribution in providing care to patients, all too often the hard evidence that can demonstrate the potential benefit to patients and services is lacking. The healthcare system can no longer provide valuable resources if the benefit is not clearly identified. Equally, evidence based care has encouraged us to review our management and our opinions based upon data that demonstrates the value of an intervention or care provided. As can be seen in these chapters we have an opportunity to set up nurse led clinics, having adequately resourced them and then, hopefully be able to identify the right objective measures to see if the care we provide improves the outcome for patients.

With the rise in chronic disease management has come the increasing need to monitor the safety and efficacy of drug therapies. In primary care the burden of drug monitoring has proved a challenge with much of the monitoring being managed in a task orientated way providing little opportunity to enhance the expertise of the individual patients. It is time now to look at new ways of working that can capture the monitoring opportunity and empower the patient to manage their disease more effectively. They, after all are the ones who have the greatest vested interest in the safety and efficacy of their treatment! Nurses can develop models as highlighted in chapter six, using the opportunity to improve patient management as well as diminishing the unnatural divide between primary and secondary care.

Chapters seven and eight focus on the need to understand the role of biologic therapies and their implications for the management of many chronic disease patients. Although the example of rheumatology is used, these biologic therapies are set to make a dramatic impact on the management of a number of other chronic disease areas within the next few years. There are an increasing wave of new therapies 'on the bench' and set to be introduced into clinical practice in the next few years. Areas such as respiratory medicine, gastro-enterology, diabetes, hepatology, nephrology and many other autoimmune driven disease areas will be the focus of these therapies. It is for this reason that two chapters are devoted to biologic therapies. The first chapter explains how biologic therapies work and the second chapter explains the importance of expert nursing practice in the assessment, management and administration of therapies.

It would be remiss if this book did not include topics such as leadership and clinical governance. Chapter ten informs nurses of some of the key components in understanding their roles as a 'clinical leaders' and follows on with an overview of clinical governance in the context of nursing development.

The final two chapters are rather special to me as the editor of this book. Individuals with long term chronic diseases become experts, over time and illness transition, and yet in the busy healthcare environment the patient's perspective can sometimes be overlooked. In Chapter eleven three individuals provide a personal reflection on coming to terms with their disease. The stories demonstrate the need to understand the complex inter-related factors that affect the individual's ability to cope with their disease and the daily consequences of chronic illness.

The final chapter – working with patient and professional organisations is one that should be invaluable to nurses. The chapter provides insights into political lobbying and the benefits of working together with combined strategies to improve care and promote the general understanding of chronic diseases and the structures that need to be in place to support management.

Collaborative working as a member of the nursing profession within the wider community of professional and patient groups is a rewarding and empowering experience, allowing personal and professional development.

In conclusion, I would like to thank the authors of the contributed chapters who have been brilliant in providing a wealth of expertise enabling this book to have a depth and breadth of knowledge that I believe will be invaluable to aspiring nurses within the field of chronic disease care.

Susan Oliver
March 2004

Acknowledgements

There are far too many individuals I would like to thank but one or two I must name...

Most importantly for the brilliant patience, love and support that Mike and all my family have provided. The North Devon Hospital Library, Bobbe my voluntary clerical officer and the nursing team.

I also owe a special tribute of thanks to the wider community of rheumatology – to the patients and healthcare professionals who I have had the pleasure of working alongside and have helped me develop my love of rheumatology.

Thanks also go to the great team who contributed to this book.

Contributors

Ailsa Bosworth, Chair of the National Rheumatoid Arthritis Society

Jill Bryne MSc, SCM, RN, Deputy Director of Nursing & Midwifery, Head of Clinical Governance, Stockport NHS Trust, Stepping Hill Hospital, Cheshire

Georgina Clark DPSN, MSc, BSc, RGN, Head of Nursing & Clinical Governance, Stockport NHS Trust, Division of Surgery, Stepping Hill Hospital, Cheshire

Patricia Cornell BSc (Hons), RGN, Senior Rheumatology Practitioner, Poole Hospital NHS Trust, Dorset

Janet Cushnaghan MSc, MCSP, Rheumatology Department, Lymington Hospital, Hants

Sarah Hewlett PhD, MA, RGN, RM, Arthritis Research Campaign Senior Lecturer in Rheumatology Health Professions, Academic Rheumatology, University of Bristol, Bristol Royal Infirmary, Bristol

Jackie Hill PhD, MPhil (Dist), RN, FRCN, Arthritis Research Campaign Fellow, Clinical Pharmacology Unit, Chapeltown Road, Leeds

Diane Home MSc, RGN, Consultant Nurse, West Middlesex University Hospital, London

Janice Mooney MSc, BSc (Hons), DMS, RGN, Lecturer/Practitioner, Rheumatology Department, Norfolk & Norwich University Hospital, Norwich

Susan M Oliver MSc, RGN, Independent Rheumatology Nurse Specialist, North Devon

Alan Pollard MA, BA (Hons), RN, Clinical Nurse Specialist Rheumatology, Leeds Teaching Hospital Trust, Leeds General Infirmary, Leeds

Sarah Ryan PhD, MSc, BSc, RGN, Consultant Nurse, Staffordshire Rheumatology Centre, Haywood Directorate, Locomotor Division, Staffordshire

David GI Scott MD, FRCP, President of the British Society for Rheumatology, Norfolk & Norwich University Hospital, Norwich

John Skinner North Devon

Jane Tadman Press Officer, Arthritis Research Campaign, Derbyshire

Cath Thwaites RGN, Dip Nurse, ONC, Lecturer in Rheumatology Nursing, Department of Nursing, Keele University, Staffordshire

Natalie Williams North Devon

Chapter 1

An overview of developing a chronic disease nursing service

Susan Oliver

Introduction

It is important to clarify that, although this chapter focuses on developing a chronic disease service based on the nursing perspective, the core principle running through chronic disease management is that of multi-disciplinary teamworking. It is therefore not explicitly stated but taken as an essential prerequisite throughout the book that collaboration and communication with the team form the first part of any discussion on the provision of care for patients with a chronic disease.

The aim of this chapter is to provide an overview of the key components that are needed to support a nursing service in chronic disease management. It includes the professional, managerial and practical aspects that need to inform any decision making. The chapter should provide the nurse with some of the 'tools' needed to enhance the development proposal. Many of the issues discussed are based on the information needed to 'set out' a case and how these steps need to be taken. Nurses may be fortunate enough to have role models and managers who will support an initiative and aid their pathway through the process; this will help greatly but is not always guaranteed. Nurses engaged in providing care can often see the need for change but find the process of making a change frustrating and complex. Vision alone may not be enough. A significant factor in implementing change has to be the sharing of ideas, but the most important factor is being prepared for a difficult path ahead. It may take much longer to convince others of the vision.

The overall philosophy of chronic disease management focuses on patient empowerment and user involvement in decision making. This chapter outlines some of the issues relating to chronic disease management from the perspective of those charged with implementing the changes. One aspect of this will be how to understand the agendas and difficulties experienced when submitting a nursing proposal to support or recognize the 'needs' of patients within the context of the wider health-care provision. In the discussions, essential health agendas and supporting evidence will be highlighted.

This chapter will:

- Introduce the principles of chronic disease management planning.
- Describe nursing development in the context of providing care in a specialized field.
- Provide an overview of healthcare structures.
- Provide the practitioner with 'tools' to support decision making.

Fostering excellence

The expertise of the specialist nurse will be that of fostering a philosophy of excellence across all healthcare settings. The nurse at the bedside is responsible for providing and co-ordinating inpatient care, and the specialist nurse should be an easily accessible link between the patient's home environment and that of other healthcare professionals in all settings. In many cases, the specialist nurse–patient relationship will have been formed at, or soon after, the time of diagnosis. This caring relationship will develop over time and illness transition. Excellence in providing continuity of care can thrive only if it encompasses the cascading of knowledge and skills to the wider healthcare teams, allowing an empowering relationship to grow between patient and healthcare professionals.

So it is clear that the way forward requires a multidimensional approach to improving patient care. It is not only about providing the right sort of care, but also collating the data, researching the evidence and then leading the way in inspiring change. Cascading knowledge and skills are an essential prerequisite for the specialist nurse. The value of the role relies on demonstrating a wide range of abilities to inform and improve care not based purely on the nurse–patient relationship. The difficulty will be in juggling all the essential aspects of the role while providing inspiration with limited opportunities to develop an experienced nursing workforce.

Specialist nurses will need to focus not only on the specific skills that may be required for increasing responsibilities, but more importantly on the personal attributes which encompass high quality nursing practice.

The key qualities essential to the role of the nurse are empathy, maturity, teamwork, communication and flexibility, and although there is a need for additional management expertise these should be balanced with developing the core qualities of providing holistic care. The attributes of the specialist nurse or advanced practitioner need to be cultivated and supported to enable each individual to extend and develop not only within their professional role but in their abilities to improve patient care across all organizational boundaries. With this in mind it is necessary to look at where the future specialist or advanced practitioners are coming from. How do we provide the opportunities for nurses to develop the skills needed to fulfil an encompassing role that informs and supports the development of the empowered patient negotiating their pathways through healthcare? Nurses need to be proactive and forward thinking, specifically in the development of service provision and nursing resources.

The wider healthcare team and patient empowerment

Many trusting nurse–patient relationships are formed when providing personal care to patients. This leads the way to enhancing a closer psychological relationship. However, workforces have changed, and it is widely acknowledged that a significant amount of care is now performed by healthcare assistants. Increasingly this 'wider' healthcare team includes colleagues working in primary care. Chronic disease patients will meet many different healthcare professionals from phlebotomists to outpatient staff, practice and community nurses, and members of the wider multidisciplinary team. The general philosophy of empowerment and developing a therapeutic relationship needs to be reinforced and supported every time the patient is in contact with various members of the healthcare team. As a senior nurse, an integral part of care is that of supporting other members of the healthcare team in recognizing the benefits of patient empowerment and identifying ways to demonstrate the value to the patient's experience.

In the past, healthcare has failed to recognize fully the immense knowledge and expertise patients have in managing their daily lives in the context of their chronic disease. Today, it is recognized that patients are experts in their field and their 'voices' are increasingly powerful in terms of service development. The Commission for Health Improvement (CHI) reviews standards of care in a range of ways, but probably one of the most informative is that of following the 'patient's journey' through healthcare. The principle of following the patient's journey highlights the unnatural barriers to providing healthcare at the same time as fully recognizing 'patient need' (Department of Health, DoH, 2001b)

The patient, and organizations that represent patient groups, should be consulted, not only for their ability to mould the service provision towards their needs but also because of their expertise in the lay perspective on the disease (DoH, 2003b). The Primary Care Trusts (PCTs) will not consider commissioning services that fail to demonstrate the view of the patient or the role of primary care in ensuring continuity of care.

Patients want to have confidence in the provision of care and to believe that they are an active participant in decisions about their care. It has to be remembered that the individual person's previous experiences will set the framework for how they will cope and communicate their needs as they set out on a new pathway managing their disease and the daily consequences of having a chronic illness. This includes coping with various illness 'crises', often on their own, at home with minimal healthcare support on a day-to-day basis.

The increasingly complex and technical nature of healthcare interventions, together with the difficulties in accessing their general practitioner, can leave many patients with long-term incurable conditions feeling that there is 'little hope or value' in their frequent attempts to seek 'specialist advice or support' from healthcare teams (Oliver, 2001). A wealth of research has highlighted the range of difficulties and emotions that form the patient's perspective about seeking healthcare support at times of chronic illness exacerbations (Bury, 1988; Corbin and Strauss, 1988; Kleinman, 1988; Gerhardt, 1990; Blaxter, 1992). From these initial discussions a picture should be developing of some of the social and psychological issues that need to be considered when planning a service development.

The patient's point of view

In recent years, some established practices have been questioned and found wanting, none more so than the traditional concept of 'care', with the patient as a passive recipient. At the same time, nurses and other healthcare professionals have advanced their skills and expertise in supporting the concept of empowerment for patients. The increasing emphasis on patient involvement is now at the centre of healthcare decision-making (Ryan and Oliver, 2002), and the paternalistic approach to care is, at last, no longer supported or sustainable.

It is interesting to reflect that the current agenda for change has been driven not only by the wish to empower the patient but also by the need to reduce the huge burden of chronic disease management by improving patient self-management strategies (DoH, 2001b). The Patient's Charter developed a 'dependent' approach to care that left many users recognizing their 'rights' within the Charter without recognizing the individual's responsibility to support the effective use of resources (DoH, 1989).

Healthcare providers have had to recognize the fact that the growth in the elderly and chronic disease populations will require increasing resources in the long term. Yet the ability to provide high-quality care for a growing number of patients is compromised by the shortage of trained healthcare professionals and finite resources available to implement care. The shortage of nurses and other trained healthcare professionals also presents a challenge to implementing change. A flexible and patient-centred workforce will require dynamic leadership and nursing is in a good position to effect these changes.

The patient is probably the nurses' most powerful ally in improving services. The nurse–patient relationship is one of strength and shared ideals. It can often begin with intimate personal care or advice relating to the patient's disease and the resulting social and psychological support needed at vulnerable times. This, combined with a strong principle of the nurse as patient advocate, forms a unique and strong bond that builds over time and illness transition. The nurse's main focus is on the patient's perspective of their disease and how to aid their coping. Yet nurses can be protective of this relationship and often fail fully to recognize the power of the 'patient's voice'. Fortunately in recent years the patient is being given a powerful voice in healthcare planning and provision of care (DoH, 2001b).

The Commission for Health Improvement expects to see a strong user involvement and will seek to explore patients' views. These views and how they can be included in healthcare strategy will vary according to the healthcare provider or hospital trust, but some examples include the following:

- Patient groups to review patient information leaflets prior to publication
- Development of patient networks. This includes areas in chronic disease where a number of support groups have joined together to have a combined and more powerful 'patient voice'.
- Links to large organizations that represent groups of patients, e.g. Arthritis Care.
- Voluntary clerical or clinic officers.
- Independent patient support groups set up to support a local need.
- Patient group representatives on trust management boards.

- Support groups and informal networks in fund raising and providing lay telephone support to patients.
- A patient representative nominated to attend planning meetings.
- Many patient groups join together with like-minded patient groups or professional organizations (for example, Arthritis and Musculoskeletal Alliance (ARMA) or the British Lung Foundation for respiratory diseases). These alliances can have a significant impact when working as a combined force to lobby Parliament with the aim of changing government policy. Work undertaken by the British League Against Rheumatism (BLAR), now called ARMA, has resulted in a document that sets out standards of care based on a consensus approach to best practice (BLAR, 1997).

Working with specific patients groups has advantages and disadvantages, depending on how organized the group is and whether they can demonstrate a consensus or a strong 'patient voice'. It is also important to remember that some patient groups are quite large and may be more skilled in representing their views than others. Each patient group, speciality, PCT or government body will have its own perspective on the issues and each of these groups will be competing for a slice of the 'funding cake'.

The culture for change

There is no doubt that, as nurses, we are now in exciting, yet challenging times. The culture is now ready for the development of chronic disease services that ensure a philosophy of 'empowerment' for all patients. The emphasis on a caring, holistic relationship has placed the nurse in the position of key worker in developing a strategy for improving care for those with chronic diseases. Yet nursing has undergone numerous transitions and 'reforms' and, although it will continue to do so, we need to ensure that changes encompass the essential essence of care that supports the nurse–patient relationship, based on a holistic approach to care (DoH, 2001c). The urgent need for changing roles in nursing has meant that policy and legislation have occasionally lagged behind daily clinical practice. In an attempt to clarify what defined nursing in the context of current healthcare provision, the Royal College of Nursing (RCN) published *Defining Nursing*. This defined nursing as: 'The use of clinical judgement in the provision of care to enable people to improve, maintain, or recover health, to cope with health problems, and to achieve the best possible quality of life, whatever their disease or disability, until death' (RCN, 2003b).

The test for the future is how well nurses can continue to make developments that will improve care yet have a clear vision of what constitutes a 'new philosophy of caring'.This is particularly pertinent when many of the new developments encompass what used to be considered the domain of the doctor. These caring activities will be subject to scrutiny as changes are implemented. For nurses there will be a particular interest in the changes that may affect the nurse–patient relationship.

The new culture emphasizes the need for nurses to develop their leadership skills and stay at the forefront of healthcare services. Nurses will need to be creative and responsive, working as 'change agents' pioneering new roles, yet be guided by their professional principles. This sounds easier than it is. To understand what we mean by 'principles' we have to question the nature of the nursing professionalism and the wider changes of role expansion. The Nursing and Midwifery Council (NMC) recognizes these difficulties in its *Code of Professional Conduct* (NMC, 2002b). Some principles of being a nurse are not simply a matter of acquiring knowledge or skills, but must include attitudes and values relevant to being part of a professional body.

Nursing – the changing workforce

The healthcare assistant

In discussing the principles of nursing it is important to recognize not only our own changing boundaries and constraints, but also those of the workforce that supports us, such as the healthcare assistant. Nursing needs to recognize that some caring activities provided in the past are no longer the total domain of the trained nurse and cannot be as the nursing role continues to be extended. The healthcare assistant role was developed first to enhance the ability of the trained nurse in working more autonomously, and second to reduce the overall nursing costs. This is chiefly due to the lack of expert nurses and the need to focus on providing increasingly complex care at the same time as co-ordinating the overall provision of care within a team structure. Although these caring activities still encompass key aspects of nursing care, they are increasingly being delegated to healthcare assistants. The NMC has highlighted a wide range of developments that employers are asking healthcare assistants to undertake, often requiring specific training (see www.nmc-uk.org). The NMC states: 'the Council has recognised that the registered practitioners require support in their work' but goes on to stress the responsibility of the practitioner to:

'ensure that all actions carried out under their responsibility have met the standards set by the regulatory body' (www.nmc-uk.org, 2002).

Yet healthcare assistants continue to increase their knowledge and expertise. In the context of nursing responsibilities and supervision of healthcare assistants, it is important to clarify the difference between a 'system' responsibility and 'action' responsibility. The system is a service (for example, the NHS) and the structured frameworks that are imposed on that individual to work within. If a system of working is defective, then the nurse, as a competent professional, would be subject to scrutiny for their role in supporting a system that failed. However, the failing of a healthcare assistant to perform their duties within an identified procedure and role would not be the responsibility of the trained nurse unless they actually condoned or supported inappropriate practice. The registered nurse would not be held responsible for an untrained member of staff undertaking a wrongful act. On the other hand, it is the responsibility of the nurse to demonstrate acceptable levels of supervision, ensuring that the healthcare assistant is given appropriate support and is competent to undertake the task requested (Hunt and Evans, 1994). The development of training schemes for healthcare assistants has enabled a structured programme of learning that provides an effective educational pathway based on the clinical needs of the service. The National Vocational Qualifications (NVQs) provide an excellent framework for healthcare assistants to develop their expertise. NVQs can be achieved at level one, two or three.

Specialist nursing

So do we have our own house in order? Probably not. Although there are important distinctions to be made between practising within a speciality and being a nurse specialist, there remains intense debate about how to document clearly and develop roles according to clearly defined and measurable standards (RCN, 2003b).

Why is the definition of an advanced or higher level of practice relevant when aiming to review and develop care for chronic disease patients? The overall provision of care, together with the ability to develop and maintain excellence, relies on trusting relationships between healthcare professionals and the patient. Equally, in the light of clinical governance, clarity in levels of expertise and responsibility of staff must be demonstrated to employers, as well as consumers of healthcare. We cannot allow assumptions to be made about our competencies based on a title.

The earliest recognition of 'specialization' in nursing in the UK came in 1919. This Nurses Registration Act identified four major specialities – sick children, mental nursing, care of the mentally handicapped and fever nursing (Dimond, 1994). The United Kingdom Joint Board of Clinical Nursing Studies was formed in 1970 to respond to the need for more 'specialized' courses for nurses (Castledine, 1994). In the early phases of clinical specialism, Castledine was instrumental in setting out to identify the essential components of the specialist or advanced practice role (Castledine, 1999). This was followed very quickly by the increasing acceptance of a need for a more 'academic' focus to specialism. These developments went hand in hand with the expansion of the role of nursing in general (Castledine, 1994).

Specialist nursing - setting a 'standard'

The Professional regulatory body preceding the NMC was the UKCC. In 1992 the UKCC document *The Scope of Professional Practice* attempted to clarify the issue of role development, stating that the terms 'extended' or 'extending roles' were rejected as limiting rather than extending the parameters of practice. *The Scope of Professional Practice* initially led to professional and legal concerns about this new ethic of openness towards evaluating competencies (UKCC, 1992). How were standards and competencies to be monitored? To some the working of the UKCC was seen to be ahead of the medical regulatory body, the General Medical Council (GMC) in developing an ethic of openness (Hunt, 1994). The UKCC (2002) stated it was for the individual practitioner to recognise their competencies and develop their expertise according to changing circumstances.

The door had been opened to wide-ranging developments in nursing expertise – it remained to be seen at that time whether the developments would encompass the 'holistic' aspect of nursing or generate a new technical doctor's assistant.

Excitingly, the opportunities afforded by the new code of conduct have enabled nurses to truly evaluate their expertise and find new ways of working that encompass the holistic nature of care. In 1993, the UKCC defined specialist nursing practice as:

> Practice for which the nurse is required to possess additional knowledge and skill in order to exercise a higher level of clinical judgement and discretion in clinical care and to provide expert clinical care and leadership, teaching and support to others.

In essence, the qualities required have been distilled into six key components (UKCC, 1993):

- clinical management
- leadership
- standard setting
- quality assurance
- audit
- practice development and research.

The emergence of clinical governance and the rapid expansion of nursing roles, together with a wide range of 'nursing titles', drove the need to have a clearer focus on the essential components of the 'advanced' practitioner. The UKCC's statutory responsibility was to protect the public. It was acknowledged by the UKCC that there was a need to address the variation in specialist and nurse practitioner roles and it set out to clarify the confusions in defining 'advanced' practice (Jeyasingham, 1999).

Extensive consultation led on to the pilot project to evaluate 'higher level of practice'. In 1999, a pilot project was carried out to test a proposed regulatory framework for 'higher level of practice'. The results of this project were published (UKCC, 2002).

The individual practitioner had to demonstrate their expertise using a range of supporting evidence. In essence, the pilot project evaluated seven standards that nurses needed to achieve (Table 1.1). They identified two levels of practice beyond the point of registration: advanced and specialist.

It remains to be seen how these standards will form the core regulatory framework for 'advanced' or 'higher level of practice'. Although these standards are robust and encompass a detailed analysis of the individual practitioner's role, it is the individual pieces of evidence presented in support of these standards that show the real nature of the empathetic and caring aspect of the nurse's role. However the process requires detailed documentation and evaluation processes.

It appears that the proposed new pay structures set out in *Agenda for Change* (DoH, 2003d) have included some of the principles used to define skills and competencies set out in the 'higher level of practice' pilot scheme.

Table 1.1 Seven standards set out in the higher level of practice pilot project

1 Providing effective healthcare
  • Nine subsets to this topic

2 Leading and developing practice
  • Six subsets to this topic

3 Improving quality and health outcomes
  • Eight subsets

4 Innovation and changing practice
  • Three subsets

5 Evaluation and research
  • Three subsets

6 Developing self and others
  • Four subsets

7 Working across professional and organizational boundaries
  • Five subsets

Source: UKCC (2002)

Succession planning

The need to evaluate the individual practitioner goes hand in glove with the need to know where the next 'clinical nurse specialist' is coming from. Don't be fooled into believing that advertising will bring a ready-made specialist or that the manager will naturally recognize the need for an additional specialist nurse! As specialists we need to be inspiring and develop leadership skills and opportunities for nurses who have an interest in improving patient care. A single-handed clinical nurse specialist is likely to stay one, unless they have the ability to inspire other nurses. The formal term for this is 'succession planning'. Succession planning focuses on the view that, as clinical leaders, nurses will always be moving forward in the development of the service and the specialist role. To move forward, nurses need to have a confident workforce coming up from behind. The support and supervision should be based not purely on the clinical aspects but on those managerial and professional skills that make the individual an effective leader and role model. Experienced nurses will be serving their nursing colleagues well if they start the process early, enhancing their expertise and allowing others the opportunity to develop with specific support and supervision.

In the current climate of nursing shortages, the lack of experienced nurses to take up specialist posts is probably the biggest confining factor to development opportunities. However, for chronic disease care, securing funding and demonstrating a need has to be tightly defined. Key outcomes need to be highlighted, demonstrating relevance to government agendas and how care will be improved as result of a development. The government has recognized the vital role that nurses have in healthcare and the opportunities to be active and powerful participants in providing patient-centred care have never been better. However, we will struggle to provide high-quality care without the expert workforce.

Modern matrons

Modern matrons have been introduced in England and Wales with the aim of providing strong leadership by improving standards and empowering nurses (DoH, 2003c). It is envisaged that the specialist nurse will be able to work collaboratively with the modern matron role to support developments and enhance aspects of nursing that improve patient care and build a patient-centred service.

Developing services - preparing a proposal

Managerial issues - the underlying concepts

If there are plans to implement a change and this change involves recruiting new staff or increasing hours or grades, it is likely this will require resources or general funding. This means that an outline proposal or business case will need to be prepared. This section provides a brief overview of some of the fundamental aspects that the nurse should consider when preparing a change or development in the department. It is worth considering issues highlighted in Table 1.2. However, Chapter 2 provides a more detailed explanation of the processes required when preparing a business proposal.

The initial proposal often forms a point of discussion and may highlight issues that the team and those involved need to review. Be prepared to have to review the first document. Preparing a detailed document focuses views and clarifies issues. It will help to form the initial views and provide a good starting point. With each proposal the nurse's expertise will develop and provide a valuable experience in preparing a framework for the next one. If the foundations of the work are strong and well thought out, it will ensure a more robust proposal and stand up to scrutiny by the business managers and PCT commissioners.

Table 1.2 Implementing change: some questions to ask

- What is the nursing provision and expertise available to implement an effective change?
- How does the proposal fit with the multidisciplinary team's overall philosophy?
- How do the multidisciplinary team view the development?
- Does the development have implications for other members of the team?
- Is the development a specialist role and is it extending/advancing current practice?
- What level of expertise is needed for the proposed provision of care?
- Are there sufficient healthcare professionals able to provide that care?
- Do the team know the patients' perspectives?
- Has the primary healthcare team been consulted?
- How can primary/secondary care work effectively together to develop changes in care?
- If there are funding issues identified, are the consequences of the change discussed?
- Have specific trust or government targets been identified in the proposal? If so, check whether financial resources have been included in achieving the targets.

Organizational knowledge

Each week papers are circulated and emails sent that draw attention to the need to focus on a specific target/agenda that has been identified nationally. These often come in the form of a Chief Executive bulletin, government White Paper, NHS Executive paper or identified needs highlighted by the local commissioners of healthcare. They may highlight the need to devolve more responsibilities to nurses and other allied healthcare professionals, or identify a set target over the next year with a specific sum of money allocated to support the change. Nurses need to scan these documents and identify agendas that fit with the patient group or proposal. It is often the case that a proposal may fail to gain approval at the first hurdle. This can be for a variety of reasons. But don't lose faith, there are also times when sums of money are made available by the government, often with little time to turn around proposals for consideration. It may be that an earlier proposal lies resting in a filing cabinet or on a shelf – it can be dusted off and, with a little work, it could be refined and brought up to date. The current issues, as well as costs, will need to be reviewed. Ensure that changes include latest policies and DoH targets or key points.

Clinical governance and networking

Clinical governance is 'a framework through which NHS organizations are accountable for continually improving the quality of their services and safeguarding high standards of care by creating an environment in which excellence in clinical care will flourish' (DoH, 1998). All health organizations have a statutory duty to work within a framework of clinical governance. The National Institute for Clinical Excellence (NICE) and the CHI also form part of the overall strategy to support clinical governance. A detailed explanation of clinical governance in the context of leadership is set out in Chapter 10.

Current healthcare provision is expected to comply with the principles of clinical governance:

- Patient-centred care should be at the heart of every NHS organization.
- Information about the quality of services should be available to all health-care staff, patients and the public.
- The framework should reduce variations in process, outcomes and access to healthcare.
- NHS organizations and partners work together to provide high-quality care.
- All healthcare professionals work as teams to provide consistently high standards and strive to identify ways of improving care.
- Risks and hazards to patients are reduced to as low a level as possible, creating a culture of safety.
- Good practice and research evidence is systematically adopted.

So what does clinical governance mean for nursing? It is the framework that forms the basis of all aspects of care and requires change at three levels:

- individual healthcare professionals
- groups of workers, such as multidisciplinary teams
- organizational.

The principles inform all healthcare professionals about the process to adopt and the pitfalls to avoid in developing or changing service provision. Some see this regulatory framework as a threat to professionalism. Managed in the right way, allowing for variations in clinical decision making, it should be viewed as a positive approach that improves the quality of healthcare and reduces variations in care. In practical terms, this means that any intervention or proposed change should recognize these frameworks. The practitioner should consider the following.

- Is the proposal based on patient need and does the service know what the patients think about it?
- Will the service be able to explain the value of the planned change to patients, managers and healthcare professionals, and the general public?

Has the project and planned intervention been explicitly and simply explained?

- How can the nurse demonstrate that the proposal will provide high-quality care? Have other centres of excellence been visited to ensure supporting evidence of good practice within the speciality?
- Best practice - where is the evidence that the proposal has a value and is well researched/audited?
- Have the wider healthcare professionals in the team been included? Has the proposal included the team philosophy of care and does the team support the overall philosophy of the proposal? Can it be demonstrated that their views have been fully explored? What about their expertise?
- Evidence? Has the proposal a potential to reduce risk and improve quality? If so highlight this.

National Institute for Clinical Excellence (NICE)

It is also worthwhile remembering that an integral part of clinical governance is the interface between clinical governance and reviews undertaken by NICE. NICE authority has an important remit to evaluate new treatments and interventions using an independent body of professionals who apply a systematic analysis to review new therapies. In recent years, the length of time that new treatments have been waiting to be reviewed by NICE has caused concern, as patients have been denied the opportunity to receive newer treatments pending NICE reports. However, the government has also stated that while awaiting NICE reports 'no person should be denied access to treatment if there is a clear clinical need for treatment' (NICE, 2001). It has also been reassuring for healthcare professionals caring for patients with chronic diseases that social and quality-of-life issues have been included in the calculation of benefits to interventions.

Commission for Health Improvement

The CHI undertakes a rolling programme of clinical governance reviews for NHS organizations. It has a rigorous process of evaluating NHS trusts using patient diaries, observational studies and interviews, as well as the usual reviews of data collected. The results of these reports are published nationally and the Secretary of State has the power to sanction special measures if there are specific failures identified (see Chapter 10).

Quality improvement is built into the clinical governance framework with a strong emphasis on the use of audit and the audit cycle. It is proposed that CHI should become the Commission for Health Audit and

Improvement (CHAI) in 2004. The new emphasis on audit highlights the commitment to review and monitor for quality improvements. The World Health Organization (WHO) has explored quality issues within the context of clinical governance. The WHO definition (WHO, 1983) divides quality into four aspects:

- professional performance (technical quality)
- resource use (efficiency)
- risk management (the risk of injury or illness associated with the service provided)
- patients' satisfaction with the service provided.

Primary care trusts

Primary care trusts became the purchasing authorities in England in April 2002. In Wales, the purchasing authority went to local health groups (LHGs). In Scotland, NHS trusts and health boards are unified to create integrated purchasing and provider units. Previously this power was the domain of health authorities. Most PCTs cover populations of between 50 000 and 250 000 people. Every PCT has a senior experienced lead nurse whose responsibility is to provide clinical and professional leadership.

The PCT directly provides primary care and community health services and commissions services from hospital trusts and other secondary and tertiary care providers. Commissioning is a strategic activity and is much broader than purchasing. Commissioning involves working in partnership with others to inform the planning of a service provision based on existing and future need (RCN, 2000a). The PCT can also commission other primary care services, for example physiotherapy, alternative therapies, etc. As a result PCTs are now the powerful decision makers in purchasing care for patients. This means that it is worthwhile getting to know a few facts about them:

- How many PCTs are there in close proximity to the work environment and the area it covers? It may be that other neighbouring PCTs also have an interest in proposed service developments.
- Who are the representatives on the PCT? Get an idea of their expertise/ interests.
- Has the PCT identified any specific target areas/groups that they wish to improve?
- Who are the nurse representatives on the PCT and is it possible to access them directly?
- Has the PCT been approached (or could it be) by a patient group or organization highlighting a specific shortfall in service provision?

The PCTs have the authority to purchase services. They are more aware of their local community needs and will be able to use their money to purchase services they see as providing the highest quality care in an effective and patient-centred manner. However, it is clear that they will remain under pressure to fulfil national targets and agendas. For nurses specializing in chronic disease management it is important to remember that PCTs have a much wider focus. They will be interested in reducing emergency admissions, reducing the time patients have to wait for a hospital admission or to see their GP, and improving blood monitoring provision for patients. It is essential to keep that primary/secondary care focus at the forefront of decision making when setting out the proposal.

Clinical supervision and networking

The use of networking and clinical supervision can have immense value when trying to identify strengths and weaknesses of professional issues and possible service developments. Clinical supervision forms part of the clinical governance framework, and should improve professionals' expertise and quality of care by supporting staff using a robust yet discreet framework that enables reflection and openness of personal knowledge and competencies, and identifies ways of resolving difficult professional issues using peer support. There are various models of clinical supervision (e.g. one-to-one or group supervision), but all models require management support to ensure adequate time and effective implementation of identified problems (McSherry et al., 2002).

Networking is the art of exchanging information, contacts and experiences for professional or social purposes. Hunt et al. (1983) looked at the professional aspects of networking and described it as 'high level group process, a creative thinking group'. In Kitson's view (1993) networks often develop at times of challenge or adversity when there is a recognition of mutual threat. From the professional point of view, networking can be an extremely rewarding process, sharing guidelines, pathways and potential opportunities to service development based on others' experiences. The often-repeated phrase 'no need to reinvent the wheel' applies in this context too. From the planning point of view, Kitson (1993) offered some guidelines for developing network links or more formal networking groups (Table 1.3).

There are a number of ways of moving forward with developments using various forms of networking opportunities. If it is a large project and the implications of the change are significant, a networking group may be the answer. However, smaller, more specific changes may need a

Table 1.3 Networking dos and don'ts

DO

• Wait for the right time
• Agree on aims and objectives
• Select members carefully and check commitment
• Cascade activities and delegate
• Thank participants

DON'T

• Try to speed things up
• Elect friends to the group without knowing their expertise/commitment
• Use others' network philosophies or aims
• Tell others what to do
• Expect results without putting work into it

less formal group but involve more of a 'fact-finding' aspect to networking. It will help to ensure that, through networking, an individual's perspective on the proposed problem or need for change is tested as 'true', and that in general the group recognizes the need for change and supports the vision or development. This means that the tools will be readily available to start the planning processes we have discussed.

Conclusion

This chapter has provided an overview of some of the issues that will encourage a wider perspective on services and the development of new models of care. Nurses are 'change agents' and it is fair to say that, although we have the enthusiasm and knowledge, we often lack real expertise in implementing change based on a structured business planning proposal (Brocklehurst et al., 1999). Nurses have been guilty of ignoring the challenges of business planning, chiefly because of the day-to-day difficulties and constraints in delivering direct patient care. It is important that nurses work within highlighted frameworks if they are to find the best way of developing services for the future. The role of the nurse has been identified as crucial and there is now an opportunity to be key decision makers, charged with driving forward patient-centred care (DoH, 1999a). As nurses, we need to take up that challenge and work towards improving the provision of care to all. It will be useful to read Chapters 2 and 4 for further information on developing a service.

Questions and answers

Question: I have suggested developing community clinics for patients with respiratory disease with the team and everyone seems to think it is a good idea. Where do I go from here?

Response: Take a firm proposal back to the team. Do the preparation work, know the facts and present them to the team. Ask them how your idea will affect their practice and how they feel about the change. You need to ensure that the discussion is open and that you are ready to listen. It may well be that a few hurdles will begin to appear at this point. Once you have the initial response look at the detail and then identify how your proposed change will fit into the national health initiatives and if there any costs or resource implications. Keep the proposal alive; seek advice with all individuals implicated in the change as well as managers. Make sure that you include patients and the primary healthcare teams who may have different opinions and needs to the rest of the specialist team. 'Build' your proposal, consult widely and then be prepared to 'sell' your case. Are there people who don't really understand the 'need' or possible benefits of the change? Think of presenting your proposal to the directorate or nursing group. At all stages you may have to redesign and review the proposal. Make sure the final written document is clear and well set out, and covers all the specific care issues.

Don't:
- use jargon
- use small text and minimal line spacing
- cram the document with facts
- ignore critical appraisal of the document
- reinvent the wheel – collaborate with other specialist units.

Do:
- discuss with your line manager or business manager before circulating widely
- ensure pages are numbered and headed
- reference DoH documents that reflect your proposal's focus
- ensure team support
- circulate a draft proposal to all the key players
- include senior colleagues in the submission of the proposal
- be prepared for a few draft documents.

Question: How can nurses develop their units and the provision of skilled nurses?

Response: First, identify what the current provision of nurses is achieving. Are the achievements clearly demonstrated to the organization? If not, a review of current practice and data collection needs to be undertaken. Can it be demonstrated that the nurses already employed are working effectively, using their skills to provide the optimum in care in a resourceful way? If the answer is yes, then clearly any new development will need to be planned with the inclusion of additional nursing time. Make sure that the skill-mix is appropriate for the development needed. Look at succession planning, and identify nurses who have shown an interest and may wish to link into or develop their expertise. Find educational opportunities to support this interest. Liaise with managers to identify key initiatives that would fit with your nursing development needs and identify new ways of working. There may be an opportunity within primary care that could provide a way for a new nursing role that may reduce secondary care workloads. The final stage is to submit a well-prepared proposal.

Chapter 2

Documentation: developing a framework for practice

Susan Oliver

Introduction

Documentation, documentation! Words that often fail to enthuse nurses, yet documentation is an essential part of daily life in healthcare. The senior nurse needs to have a clear understanding of various types of documentation, not only from the perspective of record keeping but also from the national, organizational, professional and medico-legal aspects of providing the optimum in quality care. There is a wealth of documents that support the healthcare infrastructure – patient information leaflets, guidelines, policies, job descriptions, business plans, purchasing agreements, reports, bloods tests, care plans, x-rays and many more – and it is impossible to cover all these areas here.

What this chapter does is provide information to guide the implementation of various forms of documentation based on understanding a framework in order to develop practice or standards of care. The trend for standardization is discussed and particular attention paid to aiding the nurse in developing documentation based on the key specific issues necessary for good documentation. Additional complementary information can be found in Chapter 1.

The chapter sets out to:

- Discuss the essential aspects of record keeping.
- Identify the key drivers for development of guidelines and standards.
- Review the medico-legal aspects of record keeping and guidelines.
- Provide practical advice on how to implement and monitor the effectiveness of guidelines.
- Provide practical information on the dos and don'ts of documentation.

The range and type of documents used vary but for the purpose of this chapter the term 'guideline' will be used to encompass the wide spectrum of documents. It is essential to understand the differing aims and objectives of documents used in the healthcare setting. Tingle (2002) believes that, although authors use a variety of names, there remains confusion about the terminology used and what the documentation is setting out to achieve. Table 2.1 lists some of the terminology used.

Table 2.1 Documentation: terminology

Clinical guidelines	'Systematically developed statements which assist the individual clinician and patient in making decisions about appropriate healthcare for specific conditions' (DoH, 1996)
Care pathway/ Integrated care pathway/ Clinical care pathway/ Clinical pathway	'An integrated care pathway determines locally agreed, multi-disciplinary practice, based on guidelines and evidence where available, for a specific patient/user group. It forms all or part of the clinical record, documents the care given and facilitates the evaluation of outcomes for continuous quality improvement' (de Luc, 2001)
Clinical practice benchmarking	'It is a process through which **best practice** is identified and continuous improvement pursued through comparison and sharing' (DoH, 2001c)
Business case	A document setting out the background details, basic practical issues and resource implications to inform managers and purchasers of a proposal or change to service delivery. The costs and potential outcome measures are included
Protocols	Provide a clear statements and standards for the delivery of care (NHS Modernisation Agency and NICE, 2002)
Patient information leaflets*	Information that should be readily accessible to patients. It should set out a basic overview of an intervention, treatment or service provision
National Service Frameworks (NSFs)	Government agenda to reduce variations in standards and improve care using a standard setting framework of care (DoH, 1999b)
Patient group directions	Written instructions for supply or administration of medicines to groups of patients who may not be individually identified before presentation for treatment (DoH, 2003a). In many cases patient group directions will be replaced by new prescribing legislation, e.g. supplementary prescribing
Assessment tools	Generic or specific questionnaires/forms that provide measurable data (e.g. measures of quality of life or function). See Chapter 5
Dynamic standard setting (Dyss) or clinical indicators	'A quantitative measure that can be used as a guide to monitor and evaluate the quality of important patient care and support services activities' Elliott (2001)

*Nicklin (2002) provides information on key issues for preparing literature for patients.

Documentation: record keeping

Nurses with leadership responsibilities recognize the value of implementing effective documentation as a motivating force that supports team members to achieve specific goals (Beech, 2002). The intensive preparation and review process can be time-consuming, yet the investment will support and develop good practice (Rodden and Bell, 2002). Documentation can have a significant impact on:

- patient safety
- public safety
- continuity of care
- resources
- clinical research evidence
- clinical governance.

By necessity we cannot escape the vast amount of documentation that we are involved with on a daily basis. The healthcare records of a patient provide the legal document by which the standards of care are judged (Dimond, 2002). Nurses who have been actively involved in data collection for audits will know only too well that documentation remains poor in healthcare. In daily practice, healthcare professionals see a number of patients, requiring various interventions from answering helpline calls, to attending team meetings to review complex management of outpatients and then on to the wards to review inpatients.

Sometimes the daily chore of documenting can seem time-consuming and of little consequence, but each episode of patient care forms part of a larger decision-making process. Finding the balance between succinct and informative documentation and ensuring that essential details are not excluded is at times difficult. In America, a method of 'charting by exception' is sometimes used (Tunney, 2003). This concept is one of documenting significant or 'exceptions' to defined normal or standards aspects of care or interventions. However, in the UK, normal practice is that all patient communication must be reflected in the medical records showing documented evidence of care. This has often resulted in indefensible legal cases.

All documentation used by healthcare employees will form part of the legal evidence should a case be taken to court. However, patient records often fail to reflect the detail and quality of care that is administered to a patient. At the time of providing the care it is often easy to be confident about the quality of care if the patient appears well and is uncomplaining. In many cases there are no problems with care, no complaints or sudden events, and the discrepancies or lack of documentation go unnoticed. A survey carried out to assess how healthcare records were documented showed that all case records failed to satisfy the criteria outlined by the

UKCC (Devlin, 1999). Although this was some years ago it is likely that the quality of record keeping has failed to improve, particularly in the light of increasing workloads and staff shortages.

Record keeping is an integral part of nursing and midwifery practice (Nursing and Midwifery Council, NMC, 2002a). It is a tool of professional practice and one that should help the care process; it is not an optional extra to be fitted in if circumstances allow. This is reiterated by Dimond (2002), who states that 'Good record keeping is part of the professional duty of care owed by the nurse to the patient'. Accurate documentation will have implications for care and is therefore also an integral part of clinical governance and managing risk (Chapter 10).

The Department of Health (2001c, 2002a) aims to ensure not only a standardized approach to care and frameworks for the delivery of care, but also standardized organization and storage of records, use of standard consent and discharge forms, and standard tool kits to advise on the organization of medical records.

Poor documentation is frequently implicated in formal complaints and professional disciplinary reviews (www.ombudsman.org.uk). In 1993, the Audit Commission lamented the poor quality of patient information (Audit Commission, 1993). Some issues in poor documentation can be seen in Table 2.2.

Table 2.2 Poor documentation in healthcare records

- Illegible handwriting
- No date or time
- Lack of clarity - subjective views of care, e.g. 'had a good day'
- No signatures
- Delay in completing records
- Abbreviations
- Errors, Tippex used, crossing out

Good record keeping provides an 'audit trail' of the patient's journey through the healthcare system. Patient care is provided in a range of ways, for example setting nursing care plans, drug administration and team discussions to mention a few. Healthcare records are an integral part of management and decision-making processes. They can:

- inform any legal issues relating to care
- be a live and ongoing communication tool that provides evidence of management and care

- provide supporting evidence of information given to patients
- inform other practitioners of care delivered
- provide evidence of good practice and professional competencies
- provide a framework for professional practice
- support aspects of clinical governance
- inform benchmarking and care pathways
- provide an audit trail.

All of these processes require evidence of the decisions made or treatment given. There is nothing new in the need to document all these aspects of care. However, in the past, why decisions were made or what the planned interventions were may have been variable and lacked clarity.

Documentation: extended roles and professional accountability

There are three areas of documentation that should be considered in the context of role development (Table 2.3).

Table 2.3 Documentation in role development

Professional accountability	Does the nurse's job description and contract of employment accurately reflect his or her role?
Trust or organizational support	Has the trust reviewed relevant policies and supported the role development?
Department of Health White Papers	Are there national initiatives that add to the impetus to develop or support local policy (e.g. supplementary prescribing)?

The Nursing and Midwifery Council (NMC), the professional governing body, has a responsibility to protect the interest of the public by ensuring that practitioners honour their professional responsibilities. *The Scope of Professional Practice* states that professional practice 'should be sensitive, relevant and responsive to the needs of the individual patients and clients' (UKCC, 1992). However, Seedhouse (2000) draws attention to the UKCC document and states that *The Scope of Practice* constitutes a controversial set of options rather than a true code of conduct. Walsh

(2001) provides comprehensive and thought-provoking discussions around the issues of accountability and boundaries of care, and supports Seedhouse's view that the full *Scope of Professional Practice* has yet to be truly realized. The key to these discussions rests with the need for nurses to ensure they have adequately reviewed the consequences and responsibilities of expanding or extending their scope of practice and that there is documentary evidence to support practice (Table 2.4).

Table 2.4 Structured approach to extending the role of the nurse

- Will the patient benefit from the change?
- Is the development evidence based?
- How will the change work within the local area?
- Do the nurses involved have the appropriate education and training to carry out the work?
- Does the change have implications for other staff?
- Will the development have implications for other aspects of the nurses' role?
- Is the development supported by appropriate ratified documentation?
- Will the nurse have the appropriate level of support or supervision?
- How will the changes be evaluated?
- Can regular review and feedback be included in the process?
- Will the nurse be a good advocate of the change to other staff and patients?

Nurses working in extended roles within a specialized field of practice need to have a clear understanding of their role and responsibilities. To extend or develop expertise the nurse must have the structures in place to support role extension. This may require a clear documented framework, together with recognition that professionally the practitioner is working within their competencies and in the best interest of patients.

Nurse development and the role that nurses will play in future healthcare provision are highlighted in *The NHS Plan* (DoH, 2000a). This includes ten key roles for nurses, many of which will need the support of new guidance to support practice (see Appendix 1)

It remains to be seen how the NMC develops its guidance for nurses based on current changes within healthcare and recent initiatives to enhance the role of the nurse within the healthcare system (DoH, 2000a). Healthcare agendas will need to increase the roles and responsibilities of nurses in coming years to ensure adequate provision of care. How the changes in roles, titles and subsequent expertise will be demonstrated to organizations and to the general public remains an area of close scrutiny for professional bodies and healthcare providers.

Guidelines and benchmarking

Within healthcare policies, methods of preparation, data collected and even evidence-based guidelines can vary dramatically, as do the systems to measure the effectiveness of decisions. There could also be significant variations in practice within a single healthcare organization. This is where the recent changes and focus of attention rest. It is difficult to compare aspects of care administered and the data to be retrieved when interventions vary significantly. A key strategy identified by the Department of Health (2002a) is that of developing a more 'standardized' approach to many aspects of care, not least documentation. The value of this approach can be seen in the benchmarking of care achieved using the 'Essence of Care' tool kits (DoH, 2001c; Chambers and Jolly, 2002; Embrey et al., 2003).

There is an increasing demand to create and implement a wide range of evidence-based standards, and a variety of structures are used to set or monitor these standards, including care pathways, clinical guidelines and benchmarking. In essence, they measure specific clinical criteria against current practice or care.

The development of such initiatives is not without controversy. The development of pathways, standards and guidelines has been criticized as a 'cookbook' approach to providing care, and issues such as the loss of clinical judgement and autonomy have been highlighted (Tingle, 1997). A further issue is that of the practitioner who fails to adhere to guidelines because they fail to be in the best interest of the patient. How are they to be considered in a court of law? Yet guidelines are there to support the practitioner and act as an advisory document. It is therefore likely that the practitioner who fails to use reasonable professional clinical judgement in deciding whether or not a specific set of guidelines are in the best interest of the patient could be seen in a court of law as negligent (Dimond, 2002).

The development of guidelines will not, in itself, encourage practitioners to use them, nor will it improve practice (Thomson et al., 1995). Research evidence has shown that, if the implementation of new guidelines is supported by training and education, adherence and patient care show significant benefits (Grimshaw et al., 1995). It remains to be seen how effective the increasing emphasis on the standardization model will be in improving care and reducing risk in the coming years.

Standard setting

Apart from daily record keeping there are other ways in which documentation reinforces the quality of the care provided. The perceived benefits of developing standards of care have resulted in a number of initiatives to ensure that the process of care is transparent to all, and evidence based, using various standard-setting approaches. These standards include National Service Frameworks (NSFs) as well as locally developed policies. With the implementation of a wide range of 'standards' it is then possible to evaluate practice and the effectiveness of care based on defined standards. Since 1996, the Department of Health has developed a wide range of strategies to improve care based on promoting clinical effectiveness (DoH, 1996, 1997, 2000b). There are also authorities or frameworks supporting the development of standards, and these include:

- clinical governance
- National Institute for Clinical Excellence (NICE)
- Commission for Health Improvement (CHI)
- NSFs.

These authorities are discussed in Chapter 1.

Preparation of documentation: developing a framework

Once the correct title and objectives of the document have been clarified, the next step is to ensure that the same rigorous process is applied in the preparation of all documents. This process should include:

- evaluation of evidence-based practice
- comparisons of current practice and present documentation to identify changes/or additional documentation required
- decision making that includes healthcare professionals and patients
- a clear focus on the specific clinical issues or intervention, taking into account the unusual and difficult cases that may be subject to the new documentation
- the practicality (and resource issues) of implementing the change.

Clearly these issues require a significant amount of preparation work. So what are the drivers for developing guidelines and how should the process start? The Department of Health agenda for developing standards is clear and, although some may take issue with the 'standardization approach', there are advantages for some aspects of nursing care to be supported by a clear structure or documentation. Some of these include the following.

- It identifies the healthcare professionals and organizations involved in the development of guidelines.

- It recognizes specific patient groups who will benefit from the guidelines.
- It documents the reason for the intervention/care.
- It provides background information and supports this with evidence-based research.
- It describes the process.
- It recognizes the scope of practitioners' knowledge and expertise and identifies any educational needs.
- It formally documents the new procedure/care process for clinical governance and clinical risk responsibilities.
- It provides a legal document that supports changes to an individual practitioner's contract of employment, job descriptions or recognition of extended practice.
- It enables a framework to measure outcomes/effectiveness following implementation of guidelines.
- It sets the document within a time frame and identifies a review date.

Preparing proposals and guidelines: the patient's perspective

The patient's perspective should always form the foundations of any decision making. However, the issue of 'need' and recognizing a need can be difficult if patients have nothing to compare their current level of care against (Sheaff, 1996). It may be the responsibility of the healthcare team to identify best practice and highlight limitation in local service provision. The 'Expert Patient' programme (DoH, 2001b) will improve patient self-management and awareness of care that should accessed. Patient knowledge and expertise have developed through national organizations and it may be possible to access advice on patient expectations and needs through these sources to inform local discussions with patient groups (see Appendix 3).

The service provision

Preparing proposals and guidelines: the framework

If the proposed plan is to identify a 'need to change', this will need to start with the data highlighting the shortfall in the provision of care and why the proposed development will improve the outcome. When examining the issue or proposal, try to work out how the change fits in with the latest department of health agendas. Read the latest Department of Health papers and keep up to date with reforms and changes being driven at national and local levels (NHS Modernisation Agency, 2001). Check the key health websites, professional documents, national organization initiatives and Chief Executive bulletins. Many of the funding opportunities arise at short notice and finding the time to put together a well-prepared document can sometimes be impossible. This has been highlighted by the King's Fund (Coote and Appleby, 2002) as a significant problem in developing healthcare systems over the past five years.

If the plans proposed have already been identified as a part of a National Service Framework or Pathway it may be better to find out how, as a practitioner, it would be possible to influence developments or to access the development process. It may be that a particular trust is under pressure from the local community or pressure group to change or improve some aspect of care.

Try to draw out any issues that are to the advantage of the patient, service or organization outlined in the proposal. If the proposal is working on recognized needs for reform it will help the case. Make sure that government or health service documents are quoted in the proposal.

Consider the nurse wishing to start a nurse-led rapid-access clinic for patients with asthma as an example. The first step will be for the nurse to decide if this extended role will improve patient care. The process will mean a thorough evaluation of current practice and an evaluation of the nurses' professional competencies and training needs. Part of the proposal would probably need to include guidelines to support changes in practice. As a result of initial work the practitioner may recognize the need for an additional part-time trained nurse before the development can begin. There may be advantages that can be offset against the increased staff costs, such as reduced waiting times in routine clinics and rapid access to urgent clinics. A business case will need to be prepared and resources identified or applications made for specific funding opportunities (for additional information on setting up a nurse-led service, see Chapter 4).

A change cannot be implemented without a clear focus on the current service provision. Remember that purchasers and organizations are looking for ways to measure outcomes and standards of care and, in some respect, the value of the specialist nurse role. When preparing a proposal, nurses will need to set out the initial information in the following contexts.

- The patient population: if the proposed change is for a specific patient group, the percentage of the population being targeted needs to be specified. Ensure that it addresses the needs of the patient.
- Specific details of the geography that make some aspects of care unique,

e.g. large rural population with poor transport facilities, other trusts with specialist units nearby, community hospitals and primary care resources. Compare these details with information on standards set out by professional or recognized organizations within a speciality. In rheumatology, the British League Against Rheumatism standards (BLAR, 1997) together with the British Society for Rheumatology standards (BSR, 1994) form a detailed analysis of what the patient should expect in the way of standards of care and availability of healthcare professionals.

- It is worthwhile considering, in the emerging climate of primary care trusts (PCTs), whether the planned development has the potential to span primary and secondary care.

Note: BLAR has been renamed Arthritis and Musculoskeletal Alliance (ARMA).

There will probably be quite a lot of data on the nurse's own work. The first step is to collect other data relevant to the service and proposed change. Examples of the sort of information that might be collected include:

- The number of clinics held by all members of the team and the number of patients seen.
- A breakdown of specific patient group or disease (e.g. asthma or chronic obstructive pulmonary disease).
- Inpatient episodes or number of patients admitted as emergencies.

Then consider other members who will be referring to the document:

- patients
- trained nurses
- therapists
- junior medical staff
- all healthcare team members
- pharmacy/outpatient/community hospitals/primary care teams
- specialist multidisciplinary team
- all hospital wards/specific areas, e.g. medicine.

The team and the wider organizational issues will need to support any development. Try to keep the 'target' group in mind throughout the process. Highlight implications for practice and how the intervention will address the changes and particularly increases in workload or reductions in staff support (Figure 2.1).

Unfortunately, the level of information available varies between trusts. Individual practitioners are often not aware of what is collected about their services. There are some logical steps to explore in the quest for information, but be prepared for a time-consuming process. The information gained will only be as good as the data that are collected in the

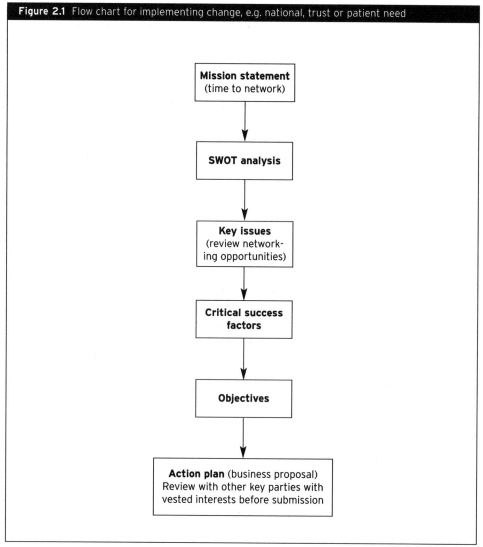

Figure 2.1 Flow chart for implementing change, e.g. national, trust or patient need

Semple Piggott (1996) set out this example of the process in the form of a flow chart. The author has modified this flow chart to take into account 'drivers for change' and the need to network.

first place. Every NHS trust has to collect data on clinics by speciality. There will be data collected on numbers of patients seen as new or routine follow-up. Information is available on cancellations and why the appointments are cancelled and, of course, they will have information on the length of time patients have been waiting to be seen. However, if nurse-led clinics are set up in an informal way and have evolved without being integrated into the trust computerized data collection system, nurses will need to rely on their own data, which may not be so easily retrievable.

A further resource available is the computer data capture department. This department collates data on the type of admission to hospital, diagnosis and outcome. It is not a very fine 'tool', because once again it is only as good as the data put into it in the first place. Information is collected from patients' notes, so the value of the data will depend on the clerking doctors' documentation plus the data capture department's ability to trawl through the records and identify other information, such as new diagnoses or other interventions. Many patients may be admitted under another speciality or consultant name and some data may be lost to the service as a result. It is worth talking to them and defining a simple search. If the nurse is able to negotiate with the department it is possible that they will set up a specifically requested search. Ensure that a specific question is being asked, e.g. how many patients were admitted, as an emergency, with type 2 diabetes mellitus from end of April 2002 to end of April 2003?

Sometimes there are gaps in knowledge, particularly with historical or financial issues, which can be difficult to resolve or understand. It may be that the finance department (ask for the manager of the speciality) or business manager may be able to help. They have often been involved in complex purchasing and agreement contracts and may be able to provide the vital information required. Use this line of enquiry effectively; make sure that there is a clearly defined question and clarify the reason why it will help the proposal. Try to be precise and focused when seeking managerial or financial information.

Having gained a broad picture of the identified need the next step is to examine the research evidence supporting the proposal. Table 2.5 uses the example of a nurse-led rapid-access clinic

Presentation of the document

A few tips will make this document much more user friendly:

- Ensure that you include a header on the top of each page. This usually includes the name of the document, author, date and page numbers.
- For clarity and ease of use of documentation ensure a logical and concise sequence throughout the document.
- Ensure that information is easy to find, well indexed or colour coded so readers can find their way around the document easily.
- If key texts have been quoted, ensure that full references to the text are given.
- Include realistic goals and timeframes.

Table 2.5 Preparation for a proposal for a nurse-led clinic

1 Review current practice	• Identify the limitations, strengths and weakness of current practice (safety, efficacy, equity, quality, access)
2 Preparation work	• Identify best practice – locally and nationally using key evidence-based research • Demographics – what population will be eligible for access to this clinic and can your intervention adequately serve this population? • How will patients access service – referral process? • Review local and national guidelines relevant to practice • Review summary of product characteristics of therapies to be used • Compare any evidence-based research data identifying outcomes against current practice • Explore issues with multidisciplinary teams/line manager/patient groups/pharmacy/current service provision or guidelines /pathways etc. • Review competencies or educational needs to implement • Explore with line manager the organizational needs in relation to development
3 Background data	• Review evidence-based data and review to current practice/ planned new model • Identify changes in workload/needs as a result of new development: (a) to patients; (b) to nursing service; (c) to other members of the team; (d) to organization and supporting services (e.g. medical records) • Cost out the identified additional needs. Be sure to include all additional costs: outpatient space, note collecting, additional investigations as well as nurse employment costs
3 Collating data	• Is the proposal or document providing additional support/ care/standards? • Have current standards been identified? • Is there general support for the proposal? • Are there specific advantages to the proposal that can be highlighted? • How will these be measured? Audit?
4 Prepare a draft document	• Be prepared for a few drafts! • If preparing guidelines that include any medicines, include the pharmacy department • Look at the organizational format and ensure that the draft document adheres to this • Write in simple terms, using an introductory section for those not conversant with specialist area. Ensure that the text is of a good size, easily readable and with appropriate line spacing to ensure ease of use. Avoid abbreviations and jargon. Get someone with little knowledge to read and appraise • Seek advice if needed from the policy and practice facilitator or education department in the organization

Table 2.5 Preparation for a proposal for a nurse-led clinic

4 Prepare a draft document (continued)	• Review codes of conduct and scope of practice to ensure adherence • Review Department of Health documents that reflect the need for change/policy/guidelines and reference • Prepare using an introduction, rationale, process or method sections. Identify competencies needed and demonstrate an evaluation process. Support with research evidence, professional guidelines, trust documentation (e.g. Medicines Policy, 2002). Final statement should be set out in a conclusions section. Highlight the outcome measures and key issues from the text using bullet points • Consult widely with the draft document • If it is a guideline or planned intervention, test the practical application • If it is a document for patients to use, ensure that it is reviewed by the patient group
5 Consultation and review	• Review comments from the consultation process • Identify changes or evidence that needs supporting • Ensure that cost implications have been supported or resource implications agreed
6 Submission	• Rewrite the proposal • Clarify and agree any resource/cost implications with line manager • Consult with revised proposal and additional supporting evidence • Plan a time frame for implementation. Plan a review date • Identify a process to evaluate practice – outcome measures (audit, etc.) • If patients are involved, review with the organization's patient group • Obtain documentary evidence of support from line manager or clinical director • Depending on the type of document (e.g. patient group direction), submit to relevant organizational body to ratify the process for vicarious liability and/or clinical governance aspect of development
7 Submission approved/ declined	• Review the paperwork • Agree the starting date • Review job description and update if new role/task reflects change in job description
8 Start the process	• Prepare outcomes measure tools • Provide early feedback to interested parties • Cascade knowledge/expertise to others. Include educational opportunities • Plan early review date to identify 'teething problems'
9 Reflection and analysis	• Review objective assessment measures • Discuss subjective views of interested parties • Are the assessment tools appropriate?

Table 2.5 Preparation for a proposal for a nurse-led clinic

9 Reflection and analysis (continued)	• Is the process working? • Does the patient/team benefit from the development? • Are the resources used efficiently? • Identify any limitations or development needs • Share experiences and reflect on practice
10 Review date	• Review strengths and weakness of documentation. Restart the cycle of preparation

Business case: managers and finance

It will be necessary to give the managers a basic overview of the rationale behind the proposal. Managers may not be medically trained and will not have specific expertise in the speciality, so make the introduction factual but set the important aspects of the proposal in a short but clear couple of paragraphs. It will gain additional interest and support if the Department of Health targets, recent White Paper initiatives or specific organizational targets may be improved as a result of the intervention. Always reference any specific information that may add power to the case

As time goes by it will be possible to have previously prepared business cases or proposals 'on the shelf' following previous submissions of work. These can be quickly reviewed for resubmission. Occasionally authorities allocate funds at short notice, with a very quick turnaround time for submitting business proposals. Read the trust circulars, executive bulletins, emails circulated. They will give a hint of impending funds and agendas, often providing vital contact links at the same time.

The essential element of a business case must include thorough costings. Business managers are adept at seeing a weak case with poor logic and planning. It is likely that the first part of the proposal a business manager or purchaser will be looking at is how much it costs and whether the proposal has been adequately thought through. The best place to access information on costs within an organization is the finance department.

Each speciality or directorate will have a dedicated group of finance staff who know the costs of an outpatient clinic and staff at various grades, as well as the detailed and more specific costs, such as how much additional money needs to be added for inflation. The are various additional or 'on' costs that the finance department would include in any proposal. For instance, if the plan is to recruit a new nurse, costs will need to include increases in salary or an incremental drift will occur on the proposed budget, with a subsequent overspend. Equally, sick leave, pensions, holiday leave and national insurance are added on to the basic salary. Give the finance department an idea of the project length, grades of staff, hours of employment and additional resource implications and they will provide guidance.

Testing the proposal

Once the aims and objectives have been clearly identified and there is a basic framework for the proposal, it is time to really test the reality of the document. This testing should include ensuring that the rationale (analysis of costs as well as logistics of implementation) is strong enough to stand the scrutiny of the business managers.

At this point the nurse must be brave enough to put the ideas through some tough appraisal. If this is not done there are two likely outcomes. First, the document may get sidelined, perhaps left on the busy manager's desk because a review of the issues, inappropriately prepared, requires more detailed time and work on the manager's part before they can respond. The second outcome is likely to be a return to the author for significant review. This can result in a loss of confidence in the idea or a difficulty in finding the time to review all the work and figures again. By the time the document is reviewed and returned to the manager, a funding opportunity might have been lost. Smart (1994) aligns this process to building a house. The key is setting good foundations. But before setting the foundations the nurse should survey the 'ground' or needs of the service. This is similar to the initial research that should be done to recognize what patient views or experiences might be as a result of the proposed development. Examine the current provision and then get a real, and realistic, feel for what the patient wants. The more work that is put into the foundations, the stronger the overall construction of the 'house' or business proposal.

Once the foundations are well under way, equal attention should go into the 'bricks' – the purchasers and patients. The completion of the building rests on sound professional expertise and skills. Although this is a great principle, a SWOT (Strengths, Weaknesses, Opportunities and Threats) analysis will help 'brainstorm' the potential pitfalls as well as the advantages of the scheme (see Table 2.6). For further discussions on SWOT analysis see Chapter 10.

Table 2.6 Strengths, Weakness, Opportunities and Threats (SWOT): some examples

Strengths

- Patient involvement improved?
- Collaborative working enhanced?
- Reduce key targets, e.g. patient waiting times or access to service

Weaknesses

- Does the change involve an increase in financial resources?
- Weak aims and objectives
- Poor audit processes. No ways of identifying improvement in care

Opportunities

- Develop the service to meet patient needs/expectations
- Build upon current service provision, succession planning, healthcare professionals' development

Threats

- Constraints on space, staffing
- A number of healthcare professionals competing for the same funding

Conclusion

This chapter has provided a brief overview of documentation that can aid the nurse in developing services. If the principles outlined are applied and the documentation is submitted only when it has been well refined, this will increase the opportunities for successful nursing developments. It can be a disheartening and disillusioning experience when what are often very good ideas are poorly presented and subsequently rejected. There are many opportunities to extend and develop expertise in nursing today, and with a business-like approach to documentation the long-term aim of improving patient care will be not only achievable but also sustained over the years.

Other chapters in this book will provide the reader with additional specific guidance on key areas, for example setting up a nurse-led clinic (Chapter 4), a joint injection clinic (Chapter 9) and reviewing outcome measures to use (Chapter 5).

Chapter 3

Telephone helplines

Patricia Cornell, Cath Thwaites and Susan Oliver

Introduction

Increasingly, the telephone has become an essential form of communication. In recent years there have been many initiatives within healthcare settings to provide patient-friendly and cost-effective services using telephone support. Although many people may think that healthcare services were the first to use the telephone as a form of support, the first such service in the UK was probably the Samaritans, set up by a vicar, Chad Varah, in 1953.

Some helplines are run by specialist nurses and others by skilled volunteers or patient organizations (e.g. National Osteoporosis Society). There are numerous specialist services using innovative practice that incorporates the use of the telephone to improve patient care. These include cardiology, urology, chronic pain management, mental health, and accident and emergency services. The aims of instigating a helpline service range from the need to ensure rapid access to services, to reducing emergency admissions to hospital and improving self-help management projects such as smoking cessation (Stark et al., 1994; Platt et al., 1997).

In recent years there has been a growing interest in providing appropriate and rapid support to patients, particularly in the area of chronic disease management (Davis et al., 2000). The aims of a telephone helpline in the management of chronic disease is to enable direct access to specialist support and specific information, to alleviate anxiety and to promote self-help (Table 3.1).

There are important issues for the development of a helpline service, including ensuring clarity of purpose, medico-legal issues, resource implications and necessary competencies required of nurses answering calls. This chapter cannot cover all the issues relating to the provision of helpline services but will provide an overview of the key issues when running such a service.

Table 3.1 Aims of a telephone helpline service

- To provide specific support (e.g. self-management, emotional support/follow-up or exacerbations of disease)
- Ensure a point of contact for specialist advice
- Enable direct access to health professionals
- Provide ongoing advice and support
- Allow patients to be discharged from regular follow-up with direct access for advice
- Reduce emergency admissions to hospital or support early discharge
- As an educational tool aiding the patient's decision-making process in managing their chronic disease
- Improve patient outcomes
- Increase patient satisfaction with care
- Support other healthcare professionals

Aims of the chapter

- Discuss the aim of running a telephone helpline.
- Describe aspects of patient expectation and satisfaction.
- Identify some of the advantages and disadvantages of an answerphone versus a manned service.
- Highlight the time and cost implications.
- Provide an overview of the legal implications.
- Describe the importance of documentation.
- Discuss the need for audit of practice and adaptation of service.

The aims of a helpline

The telephone has become an essential aspect of everyday life and nowhere more so than in healthcare. For the individual with a chronic disease, access to telephone advice can be the one sustaining and constant aspect of care in a healthcare system that can be complex and often confusing. Patients and their families may need professional advice between outpatient appointments to help them cope with their condition. Isolation, uncontrolled pain and drug side effects have been identified by rheumatology patients as the main causes of anxiety (Haynes and Dieppe, 1993). There is evidence to support nurse-led telephone consultations, demonstrating that they are effective and safe, and help to promote self-care in both acute and chronic illness (Marklund et al., 1991).

Providing a telephone helpline support for patients with long-term medical conditions presents specific and differing challenges for the nurse. Chronic conditions impact on the physical and psychological aspect of the individual's life (Kleinman, 1988). This can have an effect on occupational and financial status as well as personal relationships. Patients can feel isolated. Despite experiencing significant exacerbations of their disease the individual may also recognize that their needs do not constitute an 'emergency'. This can lead to uncertainty about whether to seek 'specialist' or general practitioner support, particularly in the early or 'novice' phase of their diagnosis (Hill, 1998a; Oliver, 2001). Equally, patients who have been diagnosed a number of years and have a long-term relationship with a 'specialist' unit might have acquired extended knowledge and only rarely seek specialist telephone support. Ideally, telephone support should reduce or clarify the need for healthcare resources and improve outcomes.

Helplines also serve as a vital resource for GPs, practice nurses and other healthcare professionals. Access to the helpline can be an effective educational 'tool', providing rapid support to key information. This can enhance collaboration, rapidly identify learning needs, improve patient care and reduce clinical risk. A discussion paper on helpline services by the Commission for Health Improvement (CHI) highlighted some key issues that should be clarified when setting up a service (CHI, 2002). These have been incorporated into Table 3.2.

Table 3.2 Framework for practice

- Protocols
- Clear standards, for example how long before the caller receives a response/what the caller can expect
- Clear information on a recorded message about what to do if the answering machine is switched on when the call requires prompt attention, and how to access information out of hours. Information on bank holidays and annual leave when there may be a limited service
- Documentation – accurate recording and logging of information
- Training and support – in listening and information giving, understanding the issues, handling difficult situations
- The patient/client group accessing the service
- Expertise – when to refer on for advice
- Confidentiality
- Consent – seeking patient consent before referral to other units/teams
- Dealing with inappropriate or difficult calls – from the worried well to threatening
- Complaints – referral processes
- Equal opportunities – how to help deaf and other disadvantaged groups

In 1997, National Health Service (NHS) Direct piloted a 24-hour nurse-led telephone advice service following the key drivers for change set out in the White Paper *The New NHS: modern, dependable* (DoH, 1997). The aim of NHS Direct was to give immediate advice and information in an attempt to promote self-help and reduce the strain on GPs and emergency services. NHS Direct is now well established and employs experienced nursing staff, who assess the calls with the help of computerized decision support systems (DoH, 2000a).

Patient satisfaction with helpline services

Patient satisfaction is a measure that is difficult to evaluate and is affected by a wide range of variables (e.g. expectations of the service to be provided, previous experiences of telephone services and individual coping styles). It is also affected by the ability of the nurse to respond adequately to the needs of the patients accessing the service (Hughes, 2003). Telephone advice relies on only one specific form of communication and this can be an additional factor in achieving an effective outcome for both the nurse and the caller. Poor communication has been linked to patient complaints and litigation against NHS services (Dimond, 2002). Litigation cases frequently quote 'lack of information' or 'conflicting information'. Communication by telephone requires additional skills, particularly as additional supporting mechanisms are not available to the healthcare professional answering the call (e.g. visual prompts such as body language).

An early study (O'Cathain et al., 2000) found customer satisfaction with the telephone service provided by NHS Direct to be high. Indeed, despite the potential difficulties in communication and issues of heightened expectation, patient satisfaction with telephone services has been demonstrated in a range of care settings (Janowski, 1995; Stuart et al., 2000).

In the management of chronic disease, it is often the nurse specialist who includes running the helpline as part of the usual daily clinical workload. Consequently the helpline service is tailored depending on the available resources. This can lead to disappointment, misunderstandings and false expectations for patients ringing the rheumatology helpline for the first time. It can also add to the stress placed on the nurses trying to run a busy service, particularly if the service has been poorly resourced.

Many units provide booklets that give information on the hours that the service functions (answerphone or times manned), additional support contact numbers (such as outpatient clinic appointment office number) and a card with the helpline number clearly printed for ease of access.

Figure 3.1 Helpline information sheet

The Rheumatology Telephone Helpline Service

Aim of the Rheumatology Telephone Helpline Service
To provide advice and support for patients under the care of Dr .... and Dr ....
in .... Hospital NHS Trust who have inflammatory arthritis.

When should you use this service?
This is not an emergency service

But it is for you to use if you are worried about any of the following problems:
- If you have a 'flare' of your symptoms that have not responded to your usual self-help treatments and you feel that you need further advice.
- If you are experiencing side effects that you think may be caused by the medication prescribed for your arthritis.
- If you experience an adverse reaction to an injection given at the rheumatology clinic. (Please refer to your injection leaflet about this.)
- If you have been asked by one of the rheumatology team to report your progress.
- If you have any urgent worries or concerns that cannot wait until your next appointment.

How does it work?

The helpline may be answered by the rheumatology practitioner or the answerphone machine. Please leave your name, phone number and short message on the answerphone. One of the team will return your call as soon as possible, although this may not be the same day. It is therefore important that you remember this is not an emergency service, and if you have a problem that requires urgent attention you should contact your GP surgery or go to your nearest accident and emergency department.

Who can use this service?

The telephone helpline service is available to anyone who attends the rheumatology follow-up clinics. It can also be used by your family or carer, as long as you have given your permission. We will only discuss confidential matters with you.

The helpline should not be used for:
- Requesting results of blood tests or investigations. If any action is required you will be informed.
- Changing appointments.
- Contacting other departments, e.g OT, Podiatry.
- General advice that can wait until your next appointment.

Other useful phone numbers

.... Hospital: ....
Appointments: ....
Podiatry appointments: ....
Therapy services: ....
Arthritis Care: 0800 289170

Useful websites

e.g. hospital website for patients
National Rheumatoid Arthritis Society: www.rheumatoid.org.uk for patients
www.arc.org.uk for patients and health professionals
www.arthritiscare.org.uk

This is thought to reduce inappropriate calls and improve patient satisfaction with the service (Figure 3.1).

Although in many cases the nurse is able to provide appropriate guidance, at times medical support will be required, either to obtain an earlier review appointment or for a medical opinion (Hughes et al., 2002). The service does need the recognized support of the medical team as it has the potential to increase their workload either through access to review appointments or time to review complex issues following a telephone consultation.

Reliance or empowerment?

An important question is whether providing a helpline service can have a positive impact on the individual's ability to cope with their disease. A study in rheumatology examined the benefits of a shared care system of hospital follow-up on pain, healthcare resources and patient satisfaction (Hewlett et al., 2001). The patients could initiate a request to be seen by contacting the department by telephone for an appointment. The intervention (shared care group) demonstrated a reduction in pain, greater self-efficacy and satisfaction. This study demonstrated the ability of most patients to participate actively in their management using a helpline service, and the ability to request an earlier referral when necessary. However, it should be remembered that there will always remain a small group of patients who fail to seek access to any form of care despite a general deterioration in their health.

A study of chronic bowel disease using a helpline service enabling an 'open' appointment rather than a planned regular follow-up promoted the concept of self-care, enabled prompt access for relapses and improved follow-up care (Miller, 2002).

An issue frequently debated is whether access to telephone helpline services promotes a concept of reliance. The term 'helpline' has been interpreted by some as encouraging self-reliance rather than independence. The key in promoting empowerment is not in the name applied to the support but in providing a comprehensive package of care, of which the helpline is only one aspect (Robinson et al., 1997). It is too simplistic to use one analysis for all patients using the service. The individual's use of a helpline will vary, depending on a range of factors. These include:

- the level of expertise and support available from primary care teams
- the patient's understanding of their disease and knowledge of self-management strategies to use

- additional contributing factors such as psychological and social issues that affect the individual's ability to cope
- clarity or lack of clarity about the purpose of the helpline
- the severity of the patient's disease – some patients may have particularly complex and aggressive diseases that result in repeated referrals direct to the helpline rather than through primary care teams
- the philosophy that the rheumatology team apply to their helpline service (e.g. clear guidelines on what patients can expect from the service or a less structured approach that provides open access to telephone advice and support).

There is a risk that some patients will prefer to access the helpline services rather than contacting their own GP, particularly if the patient feels that the family doctor or nurse has failed to recognize problems or provide sufficient support in the past. The helpline can also be used inappropriately when patients fail to get what they perceive as a satisfactory treatment from primary care and then seek a differing opinion from the helpline service. Yet it is often the case that the helpline serves as a 'pressure valve' to constraints on the service. If patients are discharged promptly from hospital due to bed crises, outpatient waiting times increase and access to primary care teams may be a problem, so it is often the helpline that will be the patient's next port of call.

This can be a potential problem and requires tact, diplomacy and careful management to ensure that appropriate care is provided despite not being able to address the overall constraining care issues. When primary care team issues are involved it is important that the helpline team communicates effectively with the patient's primary care team, consulting and informing where appropriate. The wide disparity in helpline services (in clarity of purpose and provision) is a source of potential tension for callers (McCabe et al., 2000).

Resources

In the past, nurses have implemented services by recognizing a 'need' and purchasing a telephone answering machine. The helpline service may then expand without adequate funding and add another component to the nurse's role. Often the issues of service planning are learnt the hard way after a request to management for additional resources results in a nonplussed response and questions about how the helpline was resourced in the beginning. Management and purchasers of healthcare provision may be unaware of the service provided, so ensure that it is clearly identified in the job description and outline of the nursing services. If it hasn't been subject to rigorous scrutiny from a funding point of view it might be worthwhile considering ways of demonstrating the value of the service, as discussed later on in this chapter.

When a telephone service is first launched, there may be few calls. If the helpline service forms only part of a nurse's role, establishment of other nursing commitments such as running clinics will restrict the time the nurse is able to give to the helpline. In theory, an answerphone enables effective time management. However, returning calls can be time-consuming as it may take several attempts to contact patients, thus making it less cost-effective, and it raises the possibility of sometimes compromising issues of patient confidentiality.

The time taken for the nurse to process each call, document it clearly and where necessary consult a doctor will vary depending on the expertise of the nurse, the complexity of the patient's problem and the type of disease being managed. It is also important to recognize the medical staff support required to run a helpline effectively. This should include some additional time to discuss and resolve complex problems.

A report on NHS Direct published by the National Audit Office (Comptroller and Auditor General, 2002) was generally positive, although the calls handled by NHS Direct had no visible effect on reducing NHS demands, and in particular the same people who were using NHS Direct were also accessing the health system. The service was underused by older people, ethnic minorities and disadvantaged groups, and some have questioned whether it represents good value when the cost of the service has been estimated at £45 million (George, 2002).

Telephone helplines do not generate income but are seen as an important aspect of the total service (Ashcroft, 1999). A randomized controlled trial examining a cost analysis of providing nurse telephone consultations as an out-of-hours service within a primary care setting demonstrated a cost saving to the NHS, with reducing emergency admissions to hospital and requests for home visits by the GP. To maintain such services within the community would require reimbursement to primary care teams (Lattimer et al., 2000). The cost of running a telephone helpline is difficult to calculate, although there have been excellent papers examining the benefit of the service as well as analysing the financial implications in the provision of a helpline (Hughes et al., 2002).

Although the cost analysis of running a helpline can be complex, the value of demonstrating the cost and potential benefits is vital if services are to be adequately resourced. The cost analysis should include:

- the initial cost of answer phone and telephone line rental
- nurse time spent dealing with the calls

- time spent documenting, collecting or returning medical notes
- cost of return telephone calls to patients (including an increasing number to mobile phones)
- potential savings to GPs through avoided visits
- reductions in emergency admissions and requests for additional specialist outpatient appointments.

Manned or answerphone services?

There are advantages and disadvantages to both. They need to be considered in the context of costs and quality of care for the patients accessing the service. Whatever system is chosen it will disadvantage some groups of patients more than others. It is therefore important to review the most appropriate method according to a number of factors:

- Patient needs and abilities, including functional or audio/visual impairment.
- Demographics of patient group (age, employment, distance from hospital, inpatient beds, health centre support).
- Social and economic factors that may have an influence on time of access.
- Cost implications – an answerphone will require more returned calls, increasingly to mobile phones.
- Resource issues – constraints on nurse time and ability to provide appropriate support.
- The level of support that primary care can provide to patients.

It is recognized that most people do not relish change, and patients who are familiar with a service may perceive change as a threat and feel fearful that their 'safety net' has been removed. Any change needs to be handled with care and consultation. If the service changes from manned to answerphone it is likely that the patients will not welcome this change. These views have been demonstrated by studies on changing from manned to answerphone services and answerphone to manned (Brownsell and Dawson, 2002; Thwaites et al., 2003). It is essential that the evaluation and consultation process recognizes the limits of the service and the need to use expertise in the most appropriate way. Although this may not be the optimum view for providing high-quality care, it has to be tempered with the shortage of specialist healthcare professionals and finite resources available for the service. It is difficult to predict patient views on the provision of helpline services. Patients' opinions may vary depending on:

- the level of information that has been provided to patients about the change
- the inclusion of patient views in the consultation and prioritization (e.g. changes may have been driven by limited nursing time/expertise)
- the environment in which the changes occur (e.g. if there is poor infrastructure and numerous changes are made in the department, patients may find the additional 'change' more unsettling).

Any change will be stessful to some patients. Time is needed to allow patients to adapt to the new service before reviewing the change.

Documentation and medico-legal issues

Consideration of the medico-legal implications must be addressed prior to implementation of the service (Coleman, 1997; DoH, 2003b). There is little published evidence about the services offered by helplines throughout the UK, which implies that there may be a wide variation in practice with no recognized framework or guidelines.

It is essential that there are robust methods of communicating any advice given to a patient over the telephone to all relevant healthcare professionals. In the event of litigation, all documents providing care (including helpline documentation, Kardex systems or notebooks) constitute legal documents (Dimond, 2002).

A helpline assessment sheet can provide a concise and prompt method of adding results of a helpline call to the medical notes. This will inform the next practitioner who sees the patient of the intervention or guidance provided as a result of the helpline call and may aid decisions on treatment changes, the need for additional patient education or input from other members of the multidisciplinary team. Increasingly, electronic forms of data are being collected on databases that provide comprehensive and up-to-date information about the patient. This has the added advantage that it reduces the number of administrative duties involved in collecting medical records. The method of storing data will vary and needs to be discussed and reviewed according to local policy.

The paper retrieval system can be very time-consuming and requires significant clerical support for administration of notes and filing helpline sheets in the medical notes. Documentation of helpline calls can be problematic and time-consuming but is an essential aspect of providing care and has significant medico-legal implications. In the absence of organizational policies or guidelines for telephone support, the minimum information that should be recorded following helpline advice is shown in Table 3.3.

Table 3.3 Documentation required following helpline advice

- Clear and effective method for recording telephone helpline interactions
- Date and time of call
- Name and hospital number or date of birth of caller
- If primary diagnosis known, document with present complaint/query
- Provide factual and concise information on nature of call (details of information gained), guidance provided and outcome
- Where necessary, include additional information, e.g. patient history (such as rheumatoid arthritis and recent myocardial infarction), and recent blood results where appropriate
- Advice given to caller on review or follow-up plans if problem unresolved.
- Legible writing and clear signature of person responding to call

As highlighted earlier in this chapter, the development of a comprehensive electronic patient-held record allows documentation of all details and advice given at the time of the telephone call. Electronic patient-held record systems are evolving and should significantly improve clinical decision making and communication, and reduce clinical risk.

Clinical governance and the need to reduce areas of risk have added to the need for improved documentation and recognition of the roles undertaken by all healthcare professionals. Adhering to written standards and protocols is increasingly becoming a prerequisite to protect patients and staff from potential medico-legal issues (NICE, 2003a). Such frameworks can provide additional support for nurses developing their expertise in managing helpline calls.

There is a potential risk for misdiagnosis in all forms of telephone consultation and these issues were raised by the British Medical Association on the development of NHS Direct services (White, 1998). In the case of NHS Direct, nurses are provided with an 'intelligent' computer system that prompts the nurse on questions to ask and decisions. This is less likely to provide appropriate pathways in areas of complex medical disease. Medico-legally, the nurse working within the framework of NHS Direct systems will have the support of the organization when working within these clearly defined parameters.

Guidelines for good practice have been developed by a working party made up of representatives from charities and support services (Broadcastive Support Services Telephone Helplines Group, 1996). The Royal College of Nursing guidance for nurse telephone consultation services highlights the required skills and competencies and discusses professional and legal issues (RCN, 1999).

Audit

In accordance with clinical governance (DoH, 1997), audit of practice is encouraged to ensure a high-quality service. Audit aims to show that clinical standards are met and that there are processes in place to ensure improvement.

As with all service provision it is useful to audit practice, particularly as resources are scarce and time spent supporting the helpline can increase beyond initial expectations. The increase in helpline calls prompted an audit by Hughes et al. (2002). A record book, audit form and standardized assessment sheet were used to categorize helpline calls. Demographic information about the callers and the source of calls was also collected, as were the nature and outcome of calls. The audit form enabled quick and consistent data collection (Figure 3.2).

Figure 3.2 Audit form	
Classification of calls	
Age range	0-18 19-30 31-45 46-55 56-65 66-79 80+
Sex	Male/Female
Diagnosis	RA/OA/SLE/PsA/AS/Other
Source	Patient/Relative/GP/Practice nurse/Other
Reason for call	Request earlier appt/Drug side effects/Worsening symptoms/Results query/Other advice
Usually reviewed by	RNP/Dr
Outcome of call	Verbal advice/Earlier appt/IM steroid/Seen out of clinic time/Admitted to hospital
Discussed with	RNP/Dr

The audit identified a high percentage of callers as aged between 66 and 79. Although this age group is generally retired and has more time to call, it could also be argued that elderly people need more reassurance about their condition or that this reflected the demographics of the catchment area for the hospital. There were also three times more helpline calls from women than from men. Although it is recognized that women are more likely to seek medical advice than men (Verbrugge, 1985), this figure reflects the difference in prevalence of rheumatoid arthritis between men and women. This audit form could be used in conjunction with a standardized assessment sheet (Figure 3.3), which is often of value. Use of the assessment sheet will highlight the amount of nurse time spent on each individual call and the number of calls received per day, week and month, taking into consideration the number of repeated callers. This data will assist in performing a cost analysis.

Figure 3.3 Standardized assessment sheet

Date of call ....**Time** ....**Duration of call** ....

Name of person receiving call _____

Caller: _____

Patient ☐
Relative ☐
GP/Practice nurse ☐
Other ☐

Patient name_____   M/F
Hospital number _____   Usually reviewed by
                                                RNP/Dr

Date of birth _____
Telephone No _____
Mobile No _____

Reason for call   RA/OA/SLE/PsA/AS/Other

Worsening symptoms ☐
Req earlier appt ☐
Results query ☐
Drug side effects ☐
Verbal advice ☐
Other ☐

Outcome of call

D/W RNP/Dr
IM depo ☐
Seen out of clinic ☐
Given earlier appt ☐
Verbal advice ☐
Other ☐

Signed _____

The source of the call may indicate the need for educational packages or teaching sessions with colleagues. An example of this could be an increase in the number of drug monitoring queries from GPs or practice nurses, shown through audit. In the paper by McCabe et al. (2000), a total of 9.1% of calls came from primary healthcare teams requesting information or guidance on medications and monitoring. Similarly, auditing calls may highlight the need for further patient education sessions in specific areas, such as coping with an exacerbation of their condition.

In some cases, patients may use the helpline service to request an earlier appointment because of an exacerbation of symptoms. Specific questioning may enable advice to be given on the phone that can alleviate some of the symptoms, allowing the patient to defer their next appointment or cope until the requested earlier review. One audit (Thwaites et al., 2000) asked callers what alternative form of support they would have chosen instead of the helpline. Patients said they would either have accessed their GP or requested an earlier specialist follow-up appointment. This information is crucial when lobbying for additional resources to maintain helpline services and has the potential to identify objective cost-saving analysis to highlight the benefits of the service (Hughes, 2003).

The identified outcome of calls may depend on resources available. The audit by Hughes et al. (2002) was in a district general hospital with no designated rheumatology beds. The results stated that no patients were admitted to hospital. However, if there were facilities for a dedicated rheumatology ward it is possible some patients would have been admitted.

An audit can highlight the number of patients being seen earlier than their routine scheduled appointment, with the added resource implications of fitting in extra patients into an already busy, overbooked clinic. The use of an audit can highlight the need for a review of the helpline provision or the need for 'emergency' clinics, or provide evidence to support the financing of an additional clinic (Cornell, 1999).

So, in practical terms, can a nurse providing a telephone helpline service be compared with, or complement, medical interventions? In a study in Sweden, nurse-run telephone consultations were compared to consultations in the surgery. The results demonstrate that there was good agreement between telephone advice and face-to-face consultations by either a nurse or a doctor (Marklund et al., 1991). This highlights the value of using nurses to carry out helpline consultations.

In the USA, patients have access to doctors via telephone, with doctors receiving an average of 20 phone calls per day, compared with doctors in the UK, who deal with approximately four contacts a day (Hallam, 1989). Studies have demonstrated the value of patients having direct access to a doctor. However, in the primary care setting, despite the modest improvement in outcomes, the costs were either modest or not cost-effective (Simon et al., 2000; Stuart et al., 2000).

Competencies

There are three specific ways that the nurse can ensure safe practice: the use of protocols, documentation of calls and quality assurance checks (Egleston et al., 1994). Effective assessment is essential in order to give the most appropriate advice. The use of a telephone as the only means of communicating is an area of risk, because there is no ability to use visual 'prompts' such as body language and no awareness of the patient's general demeanour to observe for signs of illness. In the absence of the ability to assess the patient visually, interview skills using 'open' questions are essential. As registered practitioners, nurses are accountable for their practice and should ensure that they have the expertise appropriate for the services they are providing (Nursing and Midwifery Council, 2002b).

Training and support in telephone assessment, advice giving and documentation are recommended to ensure patient safety (Crouch et al., 1997). However, few nurses have been specifically trained to communicate on the phone (Patel et al., 1997). The skills and competencies required of a nurse running a helpline service will vary (Table 3.4).

A nurse experienced within the field of care as well as the use of helpline services can elicit information that provides a comprehensive telephone assessment and highlights potential complex problems that need to be referred for medical review. How the telephone consultation progresses depends on the nurse's experience and the patient's awareness of the appropriate use of the telephone support service.

There are many pitfalls in managing a telephone service, particularly in the area of chronic disease management, where the patient may be well known to the nurse. This can be helpful but may also lead to a false sense of security about a patient's overall condition. Issues such as patient confidentiality can be difficult when a relative or carer phones to query a patient's care on their behalf. Tact and diplomacy need to be deployed to ensure patient confidentiality.

Conclusion

The main aims of a telephone helpline in the management of chronic disease have been discussed in this chapter. These include ensuring direct

Table 3.4 Nurse skills and competencies

- The individual practitioner's experience in running a helpline service
- The practitioner's expertise in the speciality or area of care
- Ability of the nurse to use clinical supervision and support appropriately
- The level of medical and nursing support that the nurse has from more experienced practitioners
- The availability of earlier appointments that can be offered to patients requiring urgent medical assessment
- The infrastructures that have been developed to guide the nurse in responding to helpline calls
- The nurse's ability to manage aggressive or difficult telephone calls and appropriate support
- The interview skills needed in conducting telephone questioning include the ability of the nurse to gain key information from the patient before providing advice. The key information includes: the nature and duration of the current problem, preceding illnesses or events, and actions that improve or exacerbate the presenting complaint
- Skills to support the patient to describe clinical signs (e.g. swelling, oedema)
- Knowledge of other disease processes that may have implications for the advice given
- Consideration of current medication may include name, dose and frequency of analgesia and whether any adjustments in dose or frequency may help
- Within some speciality fields the latest blood tests or results of investigations may be relevant
- The ability to access additional information that may be relevant to the decision/support provided to the patient calling the helpline
- Knowledge of when the patient's planned follow-up appointment is

access to a speciality, providing specific information, alleviating anxiety and promoting self-help. Whether implementing a manned or answerphone service, processing the calls is time-consuming and may be restricted by other clinical commitments, and it is therefore essential to plan adequately for the service.

An essential aspect of ensuring an effective and valuable telephone helpline service is that of ensuring that the patient is aware at the outset of their experience with the department of how to use the helpline appropriately. If we fail to inform patients fully about what can or should be provided using a telephone helpline service, it is likely that patient expectations will not be met.

There are arguments for and against the use of an answerphone service to record patient calls, but this is something that needs to be considered with the patient group and the best uses of resources available. There is some evidence that callers prefer to speak directly to a nurse, although changing a service provision from manned to answering machine will initially lead to a preference for the 'old' system (Brownsell and Dawson, 2002; Thwaites et al., 2003). It is not clear whether, given the option of varying resources and services, patients would elect to prioritize manned telephone advice over an answerphone service.

Audit of practice is a requirement of clinical governance and may highlight areas where a change in practice is indicated. Clinical guidance has highlighted the importance of competencies, with reference to the relevant skills and expertise needed to assess callers effectively. Training in telephone assessment and accurate documentation of calls is imperative for medico-legal reasons.

The provision of an adequately resourced and structured telephone helpline service is an effective and useful addition to chronic disease management. The increase in the population of the elderly and those with long-term medical conditions highlights the need for effective methods to support patients as many healthcare systems continue to struggle to support the increasing population's required medical care.

It is important to recognize that this is in effect a 'frontline' service that is readily available to the public, and it may be used when patients are frustrated due to constraints in service provision. Providing a helpline service can be stressful. These difficulties can be exacerbated when the service has been set up without adequate resources. The nursing time and clerical support required to manage an effective helpline cannot be overstated. Yet the rewards of providing an effective helpline can be immense and patients value the specialist support for the guidance and problem-solving abilities, and also for the empathy that nurses can provide (Wahlberg et al., 2003).

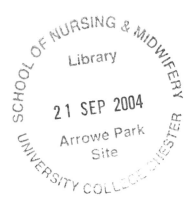

Chapter 4

Nurse clinics: not just assessing patients' joints

Jackie Hill and Alan Pollard

Introduction

In 1980, three rheumatology nurses, Vickie Stephenson, Sally Chesson and Joan Ball, met at a conference in Paris. Discussion led them to conclude that there was little or no recognition of rheumatology nursing as a speciality in its own right and consequently nurses were working in isolation with no support group or network with which to share their knowledge and experience. After many months of negotiation, the Royal College of Nursing (RCN) agreed to the establishment of a speciality forum under their auspices and the RCN Rheumatology Nursing Forum was created. This was followed in 1985 by the formation of the multi-professional organization British Health Professionals in Rheumatology. The establishment of these two organizations heralded the coming of age of rheumatology as a multiprofessional speciality and gave recognition to the increasingly important and evolving role of nurses.

In North America, nurses had been running nurse-led clinics, including those for rheumatology, for several years. Furthermore, they had undertaken research that demonstrated that a supportive nursing approach to chronic illness resulted in a better outcome for patients than a purely medical approach (Lewis and Resnik, 1967; Lewis et al., 1969). In the UK, although nurse-led clinics existed in a number of areas of chronic disease, there were none in rheumatology until beginning of the 1980s, when nurses working on clinical drugs trials began taking on responsibility for more patient-centred care (Bird et al., 1980). The supportive, educational approach provided by these nurses was highly regarded by patients, who began to request nursing consultations. By 1981, the first publications about nurse-led rheumatology clinics in the UK began to appear (Bird et al., 1981; Bird, 1983; Hill, 1985), followed by the first descriptive research on patients' evaluations of the care they received from the nurse (Hill, 1986). Since these early beginnings, nurse-led care in all specialities, including rheumatology, has grown exponentially (Humphris, 1994). This has been due to an ever-increasing outpatient workload (Kirwan, 1997), the reduction in the working hours of junior hospital doctors, and the willingness of nurses to innovate and advance their practice by accepting greater responsibilities for activities formerly undertaken by rheumatologists. UK nurses have now published several descriptive papers outlining the care they give (Arthur, 1994; Ryan, 1996a; Sutcliffe, 1999) and research papers (Hill et al., 1994, 2003a) that demonstrate the efficacy of their care. Some of these results have been replicated in mainland Europe (Temmink et al, 2001; Tijhuis et al., 2002). However, there is no published work explaining how to go about establishing a rheumatology nursing clinic, or describing what nursing care should be provided. This chapter is intended to remedy this. It is in two parts, the first providing the blueprint for setting up a nurse-led rheumatology clinic and the second discussing the provision of the complex care of rheumatology patients.

Aims of the chapter

After reading this chapter you will be able to:

- appreciate what information you need and the preparation required to set up a nurse-led clinic
- be aware of the merits of various types of nurse-led clinic
- understand the elements of holistic nurse-led rheumatology care
- determine the physical, psychological and social effects of rheumatic disease
- understand the importance of patient education.

Part 1: Setting up a nurse-led rheumatology clinic

What information is needed?

There is no definitive guide on how to set up and operate a nurse-led clinic and it is important to remember that clinical practice is influenced by several factors, including national policies, professional responsibilities and health initiatives. Detailed discussions on how to keep abreast of these issues when developing a service are set out in Chapter 2. This section focuses on the specific issues that a nurse will need to consider when planning the development of a nurse-led clinic.

The success of a nurse-led clinic will depend on the nurse's clinical expertise, knowledge of the needs of the patient and service, and the detailed assessment of the organizational environment (Figure 4.1).

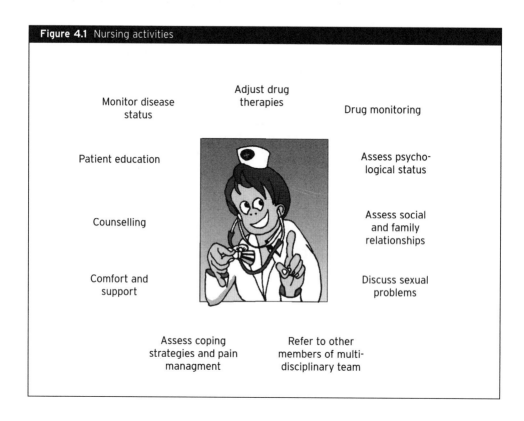

Figure 4.1 Nursing activities

Monitor disease status

Adjust drug therapies

Drug monitoring

Patient education

Assess psychological status

Counselling

Assess social and family relationships

Comfort and support

Discuss sexual problems

Assess coping strategies and pain managment

Refer to other members of multidisciplinary team

Networking

When considering setting up a nurse-led clinic, review nursing practice within your own trust and within the speciality. Look at what has been done already and what others are doing now. How did they set up their clinics and what problems did they encounter? Nurses in your own trust will be able to provide pointers on ways to acquire the resources needed and information on how to operate within the unique political environment of your trust. Make sure you broaden your perspective and investigate clinics in other organizations. Most nurses running clinics are glad to share experiences and provide advice.

Assessing the needs of patients

There may be information or prior knowledge of the extensive experience required for the intended caseload of the proposed clinic, but, despite this, the specific needs of patients in the context of the nurse-led clinic must be considered. The accepted philosophy for nurse-led clinics is that of holistic care (Ryan, 1996a) and, to achieve this, patient assessment must include social, psychological and economic factors. The needs of patients are influenced by:

- socio-economic background
- ethnic background
- cultural background
- educational attainment.

Patients from a predominantly affluent or socially privileged area might have quite different needs to those from a socially deprived area. The ethnic and cultural background of patients will influence attitudes to gender and to how they perceive and deal with health problems and treatment.

The type of organization in which the service will be provided will affect the patient mix of the caseload. In a large teaching hospital, it is likely that there will be patients with complex, rare and serious disease problems. In district hospitals it it probably going to be more generalised, but they will still deal with complex patients who do not want to attend a larger specialised unit or whose care is shared with such a unit.

An additional factor for the large or smaller hospital is the level of regular communication and the referral systems that will support the nurse-led clinic. In a district general hospital (DGH), communication may be easier and possibly more effective due to frequent personal contact and a smaller team to consult with, but a disadvantage may be restricted opportunities to gain a wide-ranging experience in a range of disease areas. In a larger hospital, where communication may be less spontaneous and there is a wider range of supporting staff to provide care, it may be necessary to build in extra points of access for support.

The factors outlined simply highlight the need for a comprehensive assessment of the needs of the patient groups to ensure that the clinic is set up with the essential resources and infrastructure.

The clinical environment

It is difficult to achieve high standards if the environment is inappropriate for providing clinical care. Consider carefully what is intended within the context of the nurse-led clinic. If the clinic will concentrate on counselling or education, it may not be necessary to have a 'clinical' environment. But if joint injections are to be administered it will need to be a highly clinical environment. Where space and resources are scarce it may be necessary to combine the two services. Ensure that, if possible, the environment is in harmony with the needs of the patients. It should be practical, easily accessible and clean, and ensure patient confidentiality. It is possible to be creative and imaginative. Use the environment as a healthcare tool, make it a relaxing environment where patients feel safe. Provide general literature about clinics, rheumatological conditions and the support available.

Ideal conditions are not always achievable, but the physical environment and initial welcome to the department will form the patient's first impressions and instil a confidence in the nursing service and department.

Assessing the organization

The needs of patients should be paramount, but it is also essential to establish if a proposed clinic is going to be the most appropriate development to meet the needs of the department and the organization. Whatever the working environment, each specific trust will have its own specific opportunities or constraints.

In a large teaching hospital, it may be that the nursing service is expected to provide an educational function and contribute to large research projects. Try to keep the service development clearly within the philosophy and remit of the department, as this can prevent a sense of isolation from the team and ensure access to senior management, making it easier to influence subsequent changes in care or policy.

Setting up the clinic

The business plan

Once you have researched and assessed the background to your clinic you will need to start the process of setting it up. The first step is to produce a business plan. This is a key document that explains what you are trying to achieve and the implications for patients and the organization in which you work. A detailed account of preparing a proposal can be found in Chapter 2, and this should be used in conjunction with the information outlined in this chapter to set out your proposal.

For a nurse-led clinic proposal the document should include the following:

- The purpose of the clinic, identified and anticipated needs of patients. Be clear about the type of clinic (e.g. general or specific disease group).

- Expected patient numbers and projected changes in workload in the next financial year.
- Justification for the capital expenditure and potential benefits to the trust and services including how performance can be measured (audits and clinical performance measures).
- Details of physical resources required (rooms, equipment, etc.).
- Practical issues related to the identified workload for the management of the clinic and work implications for other services involved in the clinic.
- Use objective language and research evidence. Focus on evidence-based practice or models of good practice. It will also demonstrate a thorough and rigorous approach to your background research.
- Highlight feedback gained from interviewing or meeting with key groups that will affect or be affected by the nurse-led clinic.
- Do not make claims that cannot be substantiated. Your plan should present an unassailable case.
- Ensure that the plan includes all the resources necessary for you to achieve the defined aims of the clinic. Be practical and realistic, but aim for the best. If you do not ask for it you will not get it and it is usually more difficult to obtain additional resources once a service has been established.
- Do not leave loose ends. If it could ever be achieved, the ideal business plan would answer every question management needed to ask.

Developing a business plan may appear a daunting prospect, but it is an excellent discipline. It will force consideration of every aspect of the project and provide a real grasp of the practicalities involved. Moreover, a good business plan will persuade those who control resources that you have the ability to use those resources efficiently and the will to make a success of the project.

Clinic administration

The need for properly resourced and effective administrative support cannot be overemphasized. Many nurse specialists and nurse consultants have been unable to provide the service they would like because of the inadequacy or complete absence of administrative support (Guest et al., 2001). Consider carefully what is required for the proposed clinic.

Practices vary from hospital to hospital and time will be well spent researching the fine details of all aspects of documentation, data collection and administration. The frustration and time that can be saved by good clerical support cannot be overstated; without it, safe and effective nurse clinics cannot be considered.

Obtaining the appropriate resources

Once the proposal has been accepted and recognized by the department and management, the challenge will then be how to obtain the physical resources needed to make the clinic possible. This can often be the greatest stumbling block and will require tact, diplomacy and, to a certain degree, shrewd networking opportunities to gain access to all that is required. Negotiation and compromise may be necessary to obtain what is required. It is for this reason that the initial proposal should document every item that is needed. For example:

- Detail the supplies, ancillaries, storage, clinical preparation areas, hygiene facilities and consultation areas required.
- Prioritize requests – identify the essential and preferable items.
- Be prepared to 'barter' for resources. This may sound ruthless but it is often the reality.
- Be prepared to share facilities. Though not ideal, it is a start.
- Expect bureaucratic obstacles.
- Be persistent.

Then, given that a compromise has been reached, celebrate and collate a list to prepare for the following year's proposal to improve on the initial resources provided.

Identifying clinical need

What should nurse-led clinics provide?

Typical clinic activities are drug and disease monitoring, drug administration, counselling, education and social care. In general, the clinics described above encompass all these aspects, although the emphasis may vary. A balance must be struck to achieve optimum effectiveness. For example, concentrating on education at the expense of other activities may result in a patient having to return for monitoring, or important clinical findings may be delayed. Conversely, a highly clinical focus in relation to physical monitoring might cause safety problems if educational needs are not met.

Specialized or general type of clinic?

Whether specialized or general clinics are adopted will depend on the number and type of patient, the nature of the department and the resources available. It is necessary to consider what is in the best interest of the patient population in the long term before making a decision about the type of service to be provided. There is no universal optimum mix of clinic type and clinic frequency – the solution can be determined only by assessing local need.

In some large units, specialist clinics run in tandem with other specialities to meet specific patients needs, for example combined clinics with dermatology, neurology and respiratory departments for complex connective tissue disorders. Nursing support for these clinics should be carefully considered and may provide opportunities to collaborate with other specialist nurses to ensure effective care.

Whatever the service being provided, the clinic should maintain continuity of care by providing access to other members of the multidisciplinary team, including a consultant when necessary. For specific complex disease groups it may be essential to run the clinic in tandem with the consultant clinic so that new problems presenting in the nurse clinic can be rapidly resolved

The gold standard would be to ensure access to all members of the multidisciplinary team on the same day in the same environment, which reduces the need for further appointments. However, as already discussed, compromises have to be made and these issues must be considered in the context of providing a high-quality service. An additional advantage that needs to be highlighted when negotiating for resources and clinic time should be the fact that audit and research work can be carried out more efficiently, enabling an efficient and tailored approach to meet individual patient needs.

Examples of nurse clinics

General rheumatology monitoring

General rheumatology monitoring clinics involve monitoring patients in relation to drug therapy, disease activity, and physical and psychological wellbeing. They also provide an environment for education and counselling of patients with rheumatoid arthritis (RA), polymyalgia rheumatica (PMR), gout, osteoarthritis (OA) and other rheumatological conditions not served by other clinics. For some nurse specialists, monitoring predominates, while others focus largely on the educational and counselling functions. Most clinics will combine elements of both.

Nurse-led clinics for RA patients in remission

Patients with RA who have been in remission for a year or more may benefit from nurse-led clinic reviews. These patients can be monitored and reviewed effectively by a nurse specialist working within clearly defined guidelines and protocols. This enables the nurse to monitor medications and disease activity as well as review important aspects of care such as patient concordance with therapy. Patients remain under the care of a consultant but are reviewed as deemed necessary by the nurse specialist or according to set protocols. The patient's follow-up care is often tailored according to their specific clinical needs.

Connective tissue clinic

Connective tissue disorders can be seen in dedicated nurse-led clinics. These can be divided into specific disease groups, such as lupus or scleroderma, or combined in a general connective tissue disease clinic. These specialist clinics should also provide a disease monitoring service, helpline contact, counselling and education.

Seronegative arthropathy clinic

These are for patients with ankylosing spondylitis (AS) and psoriatic arthritis (PA). This is sometimes a joint clinic, with the nurse and physiotherapist providing a one-stop review.

Biologic therapy clinic

Many areas have set up specific clinics for biologic therapies. These are usually run by a dedicated nursing service. This can enable the nurse to focus on the key issues of screening, assessment and preparation of patients, reducing clinical risk and acting as an educational resource for patients and other healthcare professionals.

Patients should receive specific monitoring, education and counselling for these therapies, in addition to care for their general needs, particularly as many have a severe disease and require substantial support.

Nurse clinics for medical research

Clinical trials, either in conjunction with pharmaceutical companies or providing for the needs of research within the department, usually need dedicated research nurses. These nurses often collect data and provide the education necessary to inform patients about the nature of the clinical trials, therapy administration and monitoring. Dedicated time needs to be allocated for the detailed documentation and administration necessary for research data collection.

Telephone clinics

Patients are given the number of a telephone helpline which allows them to contact the nurse specialists with questions, or problems that do not require urgent attention. A detailed account of telephone help advice lines is given in Chapter 3.

Points for discussion

Acting as the leader

Operating a nurse-led clinic is sometimes perceived as an isolated role. In reality, a clinic will involve several people, some of them all of the time and others on an intermittent basis. How well the clinic functions and how successful it is will depend on the extent to which all those involved can act as a team. The task of motivating and leading this team will fall to the nurse running the clinic and so good leadership skills will be central to success in this endeavour.

Running a nurse-led clinic involves aspects of leadership and acting as a role model. Ensuring an effective approach to leadership issues will build confidence in individuals supporting the service and the larger team helping to meet desired outcomes from the patient's perspective, the organization's perspective and a professional perspective. A discussion of leadership skills is outside the scope of this chapter (see Chapter 10).

The multidisciplinary team

As a nurse conducting nurse-led clinics it will be essential to work as part of the multidisciplinary team because care will affect and be affected by the work of others within the team. The perceptions of 'team' and what constitutes a team will differ in various settings, and the scope and range of team members available will vary. Some units include the secretarial and clerical staff as 'team'; other units have the full complement of team, including podiatry and psychology; others may not. As a result, professional responsibilities may vary between organizations. In some environments, physiotherapists and occupational therapists carry out joint protection, whereas in others it is the responsibility of nurses. An additional factor will be what individual team members perceive as intrinsic aspects of their role. In some areas, aspects of care and expertise may overlap. This can often be to the benefit of the patient. However, as a team, effective communication, clarity of roles and aspects of overlap must be clearly recognized.

Table 4.1 Members of the multidisciplinary team and relationship with nurse-led clinic workload

Team member	Principal functions
Clinical nurse specialist	Provides nurse-led clinics for patients as part of their role
Ward nurse	Co-ordinates daily care for patients. Refers patients to nurse-led clinics and receives referrals from them for inpatient or day care services
Outpatient nurse	Helps to support outpatient nurse-led clinics. Can provide help with basic nursing support for patients. Assists in basic monitoring and administration of therapies in some areas
Physiotherapist	Accepts referrals from and refers to nurse-led clinics. Provides an information source on physiotherapy matters, exercise, etc.
Occupational therapist	Accepts referrals from nurse-led clinics and refers to nurse-led clinics. Provides a knowledge pool regarding support services and strategies for patients, splinting services, etc.
Podiatrist	Accepts referrals from nurse-led clinics and refers to nurse-led clinics. Acts as an information and education resource for the nurses leading the nurse-led clinics and patients attending them regarding foot care and treatment
Pharmacist	Acts as information and education resource for the nurse regarding drug therapy, interactions, safe use and setting up of clinical services for drug administration, etc.
Consultant rheumatologist	Refers to nurse-led clinics and accepts referrals from them. Provides drug therapeutic interventions and diagnostic services. Assists in dealing with urgent problems. Provides a clinical resource for medical therapeutic requirements and approaches. In some areas may provide some managerial support
Other involved medical staff	Assist the consultant rheumatologist in meeting medical needs of patients and medical support for patients attending nurse-led clinics. May change drug dosage or advise on or administer certain therapeutic interventions
Clinic clerk	Ensures that notes are up to date and available for nurse-led clinics. Acts as receptionist for clinics. Assists in finding notes and results, and helps solve administration problems. Deals with clinic enquiries and changes to appointments where appropriate. Maintains appointment records on the hospital computer system
Secretarial staff	Type clinical letters. May be able to take certain enquiries regarding patient care
Domestic staff	Maintain a clean and tidy environment for conducting the clinics

Table 4.1 shows potential team members. It is not definitive, but is intended to stimulate thought on the interactions within multidisciplinary teams and perhaps highlight people who may influence the clinic but may not be considered as obvious members of the multidisciplinary team.

For the multidisciplinary team to function effectively, all those involved need a clear understanding of their own role and that of all other team members. Roles may differ in different settings, but the essential requirement is that everyone has clarity of their professional role and responsibilities.

Summary of key points

- Consider carefully the needs of the patients.
- Review the needs of the department and the organization.
- Identify issues that inform decisions about service provision, e.g. local, national health policy and the political environment.
- Decide on the type of clinic that is most appropriate according to need.
- Create a business plan.
- Reflect on the issues of leadership and, if necessary, take steps to improve leadership skills.
- Understand administrative requirements.
- Form a clear view of the role of multidisciplinary team and of the nurse clinics.

Part 2: Holistic care of the rheumatology patient in a nurse-led clinic

Background

Chronic disease has been described as 'a dramatic, unforeseen and unasked for life event which presents both physical and psychological problems' (Arthur, 1998), and this is certainly the case for many patients with a complex rheumatic disease. The diseases themselves are both commonplace and diverse, with some authors quoting as many as 200 individual disorders (Symmons and Bankhead, 1994). The literature suggests that rheumatoid arthritis is the most common disease seen in nurse-led clinics, but, as mentioned earlier in this chapter, nurses see patients with many other rheumatic conditions. Although the rheumatic diseases themselves are heterogeneous, from a nursing perspective they share a number of common features in that they are usually:

- incurable
- painful
- debilitating
- functionally limiting
- life altering.

It is not surprising therefore that rheumatic diseases can lead to social isolation, anxiety, depression and loss of self-esteem.

Nursing and the rheumatic diseases

The provision of holistic care for this group of vulnerable people demands mastery of a whole gamut of nursing skills, but primarily the ability to work as a partner with the patient and their family. However, it should be remembered that one profession in isolation cannot successfully manage such complex diseases, and the nurse often acts as a co-ordinator of care for other members of the multidisciplinary team. No matter which disease the patient has, the key functions of nursing care remain applicable (Table 4.2), and the philosophy should be to provide the means by which patients can live as full and enriched a life as possible, despite their disease.

Table 4.2 The key functions of nursing

- Understanding illness and treatment from the patient's perspective
- Providing continuous psychological care during illness and critical events
- Providing comfort
- Enabling people to cope with illness or potential health problems
- Co-ordinating treatment and other events affecting the patient

Source: Wilson Barnett (1984)

Nursing care from the nurse-led clinic

The nurse working from a nurse-led clinic plays a pivotal role in the provision of holistic care. The role of the nurse is in itself complex and has been defined by the RCN (2003b) as:

> the use of clinical judgement in the provision of care to enable people to improve, maintain, or recover health, to cope with health problems, and to achieve the best possible quality of life, whatever their disease or disability, until death.

This definition provides a template for nurses, irrespective of speciality or the environment in which they find themselves. The elements relevant to rheumatology nursing are:

* empowerment
* rehabilitation
* education
* patient participation.

The one element that may not be pertinent to chronic rheumatic diseases is the recovery of health, as many disorders are at present incurable.

Components of care

The key components of care in the nurse-led clinic are shown in Table 4.3 and, although this list appears short, they comprise many different facets that cascade into a multitude of different activities, some of which are displayed in Figure 4.1. Dealing with such a plethora of activities can be daunting even to the experienced nurse, and perhaps the best way of approaching it is to use a nursing model, such as the RCN Rheumatology Nursing Forum model, which was developed specifically for the task (Figure 4.2). This is based on the problems that patients commonly experience, such as their symptoms and their associated effects. However, it also incorporates psychosocial elements, and emphasizes the importance of underpinning management with patient education.

Care planning

Many patients are referred to nursing clinics for routine monitoring of drug therapy for efficacy and side effects (Phelan et al., 1992), a topic covered elsewhere in the literature (Ryan, 1997) and in Chapter 6. For whatever reason patients are referred, care planning should be holistic and comprise those components shown in Table 4.3.

Table 4.3 Components of care in the nurse-led clinic

* Managing the patient's disease
* Identifying the patient's problems
* Determining the patient's coping strategies
* Appraising the patient's knowledge of their disease and its treatments
* Establishing a care plan
* Acting as an expert source of referral

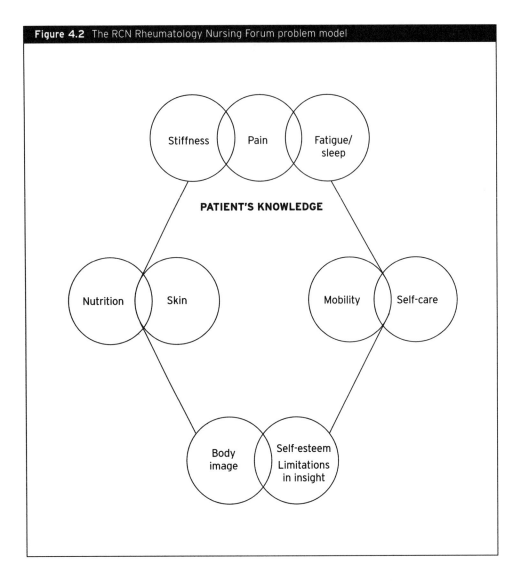

Figure 4.2 The RCN Rheumatology Nursing Forum problem model

When referred to the nurse-led clinic, patients who have never experienced care from a nurse may have little idea of what to expect. The patient may also have received their diagnosis only recently and different people will react in different ways. Some are simply relieved to have a definite diagnosis, while others are bewildered and afraid, going through stages of shock, disbelief, denial, grief, hostility, anger and finally adjustment, all emotions associated with the grieving process. The different reactions of acceptance and denial are well illustrated by two female patients recently seen in our outpatient clinic for early inflammatory arthritis. When asked how they felt when they were first told they had rheumatoid arthritis the first patient replied:

> I just felt relieved because if you have a name for it and you know what it is, you can do something about it. The doctor was very nice and told us [her husband was with her] about the treatments, you know the drugs and that. He said they had changed a lot and that you started them early so that it stopped the joints going wonky. I read all the booklets from the clinic, you know the ARC ones, and I've been on the Internet and found out as much as I can. It's important to know everything you can. I feel quite well at the moment, can't complain.

This patient had accepted her diagnosis and was ready to accept more information about her disease and treatments. The second patient was similar in age, social circumstances, diagnosis and disease duration, but her response was completely different. Her reply was:

> I was devastated. He [the doctor] told me I had rheumatoid arthritis and I'd had an auntie who died of it. I kept thinking about her and how she was old and had twisted hands. She was in a wheelchair. I thought that kind of arthritis only happened to old people and I was only 44. How could I have it? He said that I needed some tablets and I don't like taking tablets. When I got home I cried. He gave me a pre-scription and told me I had to have blood tests every few weeks. I didn't have time to go to have blood tests because I work for a living. I decided to leave the tablets and see how I went on.

This patient was in denial and not ready to move ahead. She needed more time to come to terms with her condition and counselling sessions were more appropriate in her case.

Even though both patients had recently entered the mystifying world of illness, their reactions to it were quite different and consequently the care they required would be very different.

The nurse-patient consultation

Perhaps the most important nurse–patient encounter is the first consultation. It should be remembered that identifying and understanding the patient's problems takes time and patience, and it is at this first encounter that the pattern for the development of the important nurse–patient relationship is set. From the patient's perspective, ample time should appear to be available even when in reality it is not. This can be tricky to say the least!

Baseline assessments such as those described in Chapter 5 should be undertaken and used to provide the foundation for an assessment of the

Table 4.4 Topics typically reviewed for inclusion in a care plan

Symptom management	
Pain control	Thermal therapy
	Transcutaneous electrical nerve stimulation
	Analgesia advice and review of therapeutic options where appropriate
	Pacing and prioritizing activities
	Relaxation
Fatigue control	Assessment of sleep pattern
	Dietary assessment
	Pacing and prioritizing activities
	Disease status, including haematology for anaemia
Function	
Home adaptations	Tap turners/raised toilet seat/shower, etc.
Splints	Wrist splints, sleeping splints, etc.
Foot assessment	Insoles, shoes
Social needs	
Financial status	Work, benefits
Relationships	Partner, family, friends, colleagues
Social isolation	Outside interests, transportation
Emotional needs	
Self and body image	Effects on sexual and social relationships
Psychological status	Anxiety and depression
Educational needs	
Knowledge	Disease, treatments and coping strategies
Self-efficacy	Belief that they can make a positive impact on outcome
Multidisciplinary needs	
Physiotherapy	Exercise regime, walking aids, etc.
Occupational therapy	Splints, pacing and prioritizing, etc.
Orthotics	Prostheses such as knee braces, callipers, etc.
Podiatrist	Foot assessment, insoles, etc.
Social worker	Financial allowances, home adaptations, etc.
Dietician	Dietary advice
Many others	

patient's outcome. Subsequent sequential recordings can be compared with this baseline data and it will also provide information at a later stage for an audit of outcomes from the nurse-led clinics. This first consultation should provide enough information on which to base a comprehensive nursing care plan, and typical topics for inclusion are shown in Table 4.4. The care plan and how problems are to be resolved should be agreed with the patient It is important to include information regarding:

- the patient's problems
- the method to be used to deal with problems
- the outcome sought
- the response to the prescribed therapy.

The symptoms of chronic diseases such as RA and OA tend to be cyclical and patients can experience periods of exacerbation and remission. The care plan must be flexible enough to accommodate alterations as new problems arise and old problems change or are solved. It is unlikely that the complex problems that are associated with rheumatic diseases will be effectively addressed on one clinic visit, and so subsequent appointments will need to be planned and documented.

The nursing care plan is an important document and, although it takes a little time to formulate and update, it is an invaluable tool in patient management.

Physical care

The physical symptoms of rheumatic disease include pain, joint stiffness, fatigue and limitation of movement. All of these symptoms can be extremely distressing when patients are trying to carry on their normal lives. The role of the nurse is to enable the patient to manage their symptoms as effectively as possible by providing information and patient education as appropriate.

Pain

Pain is the primary reason that patients with rheumatic disease seek medical advice (Symmons and Bankhead, 1994) and the majority cite this as their most discomforting symptom. The type of pain experienced will dictate the treatment advocated. Pain may be generalized, with many joints affected, or it could be restricted to just one or two joints. It is important to try to identify the cause of the pain, and to do this it might be useful to review the following questions:

- How long has the pain been present?
- Is it getting worse?
- Is it a flare?
- Is it loss of disease control?
- Is it due to overuse of the joints?
- Is the patient anxious or depressed?
- Has anything helped?

Having this information will help in the identification of the most appropriate method of relief. The most commonly used treatments are:

- drug therapy (including intra-articular injections)
- physiotherapy
- splinting
- pacing and prioritizing
- thermal therapy – heat and cold
- relaxation techniques
- transcutaneous nerve stimulation (TENS).
- patient education.

It may be necessary to combine a number of different measures and these are discussed in detail in other texts (Hill, 1998). It is important to remember that patients often have their own remedies and these should not be ignored. After all, they are the 'experts' as far as their disease is concerned and they will be the ultimate judge of what level of pain is acceptable to them.

Stiffness

Stiffness can be a major problem for patients. It can alter their ability to function and reduce their quality of life. It is often at its worst first thing in the morning – 'morning stiffness' – but it can occur at any time of day, usually following periods of rest when it is called 'inactivity stiffness'. The cause of the stiffness may provide an indication for its relief. The most common causes are:

- inflammation
- soft tissue thickening
- changes to the articular surfaces of the bones
- alterations to mechanical integrity
- excess synovial fluid.

Early morning stiffness may be relieved by undertaking gentle exercise on waking, followed by a warm bath or shower. Non-steroidal anti-inflammatory drugs (NSAIDs) may also help, as they reduce inflammation. An increasing duration of early morning stiffness may indicate that the patient is going into a flare, and the nurse must ensure that the patient knows how to manage this condition if it occurs. Inactivity stiffness can be relieved by frequent changes of position and gentle range-of-movement exercise while sitting. Alleviation of morning stiffness is very much akin to pain relief measures and more detailed information is available elsewhere (Hill, 1998).

Fatigue

Patients, particularly those with inflammatory disease, frequently complain about overwhelming fatigue. Fatigue is a characteristic of many rheumatic diseases and the two most common causes are:

- disease activity
- sleep disturbance.

However, patients tend to attribute fatigue to the need to exert twice the effort and expend twice the energy to carry out a task as they did prior to being diagnosed (Crosby, 1991).

Disease activity

In general, the more active the disease, the worse the fatigue. This is caused by a number of factors, including anaemia due to RA (Turnbull, 1987). It is important that patients understand this association, as they will be more likely to establish the necessary work/rest cycle that may help to alleviate it. Knowing that fatigue is a symptom of their disease often brings great relief to patients, as they can give themselves permission to rest and relax without feeling guilty. It is also important that family members know of the problem, so that they can provide assistance with general activities and help to reinforce the need for pacing and reduced activities.

Sleep disturbance

Sleep plays an important role in recovering from illness, and if the condition is chronic it may be even more important. Sleep disturbance is often caused by pain, but there are other causes, such as anxiety, depression and some medications, which are known to disrupt sleep (White, 1998). Pre-emptive use of analgesics or non-steroidal anti-inflammatory drugs, the application of splints and special pillows to alleviate neck pain can help to reduce sleep disturbance caused by pain. The causes of anxiety and depression need further investigation. Frequently, problems can be solved by discussion with the nurse, but some patients may require a specialist referral. An in-depth text that discusses fatigue and sleep and positive nursing interventions is available (White, 1998).

Psychosocial care

One of the most highly valued fundamentals of rheumatology nursing is the 'caring role'. Caring comprises both physical and emotional components and it is essential that these are given equal emphasis. When patients present in the nurse-led clinic the physical signs of their disease are usually visually obvious, in the form of synovitis, redness, swelling or joint deformity, and can be dealt with. What is less evident are the ensuing psychological effects, and it is imperative that these are also addressed.

Chronic rheumatic diseases have a global impact on both the patient and those who are closest to them. This can lead to:

- lack of self-esteem
- reduced psychological status, e.g. anxiety and depression
- problems with relationships
- changes to family and social roles
- negative perceptions of control.

All of these require investigation if nursing care is to be truly holistic.

Reif (1975) has highlighted the following problems as being particularly associated with chronic disease:

- Interference with normal routines and activities due to the disease symptoms.
- Limited effectiveness of medical regimens.
- Substantial disruption of the usual pattern of living brought about by treatments intended to mitigate symptoms and long-term effects of the disease.

These problems are brought to the fore when a patient realizes that the treatments they are taking or undergoing are palliative rather than curative, and this is reinforced if they go into a flare. Flares can be very stressful, reminding the patient of the fragility of their physical status, and this can impact negatively on mood and feelings of control, often resulting in social isolation. Uncertainty is enhanced in the 'novice' patient as they are unfamiliar with their disease and their expectations do not match their experience. For example, a patient starts disease-modifying anti-rheumatic drug therapy with the expectation that their symptoms will improve. Three weeks later there is no change – the patient's experience does not match their expectation and so they become more uncertain, anxious and/or depressed and afraid.

At this novice stage, provided they have accepted their diagnosis, patients need to learn about their disease and its treatments, and they usually express their readiness by seeking information. A patient will feel less threatened and more in control if they know what to expect. Written information is a very useful adjunct to verbal explanation, as it can be kept for future reference and also shared with others. This stage of the patient's illness journey can be likened to the first of the three stages on the road to mastery (Table 4.5) derived from research undertaken using in-depth interviews with women with RA (Shaul, 1995). A series of questions has been devised that enable the nurse to decide which stage the patient has reached (Table 4.5) and so determine the necessary solutions (Ryan, 1998).

Anxiety and depression

There is a high prevalence of anxiety and depression in people with RA. It has been suggested that 21–34% of patients are affected (Creed, 1990), with depression being the more common of the two (Parker and Wright, 1995). These levels are similar to those found with other chronic disease patient groups (Hawley and Wolfe, 1988). Both anxiety and depression have been shown to respond to discussion with patients about their fears and anxieties, and this is well demonstrated in a study of outcome from a nurse-led rheumatology clinic (Hill et al., 1994). Another proven intervention is patient education. A literature review of 76 studies of arthritis patient education showed that depression reduced in nine of the 17 studies in which it was measured. Similarly, levels of anxiety reduced in five of the six studies in which it was measured (Lorig et al., 1987).

Pain

Pain has been shown to influence psychological status. A study of 400 patients with RA, who were followed over a four-year period, found that those with increased levels of pain also tended to have higher levels of anxiety and depression (Hawley and Wolfe, 1988). Moldofsky and Chester (1970) also suggested a link between pain and depression in a study in which they were able to delineate depression into two specific

Table 4.5 Guidance on assessing the stages of mastery over arthritis - Stages of Mastery

1 Becoming aware - the initial stage

The patient becomes aware that the symptoms are not going away or they are increasing and interfering with everyday life. The first few years are the worst as patients struggle with the physical effects that impact on their emotional wellbeing

Assessment questions:
- What symptoms does your arthritis cause?
- What does your arthritis prevent you from doing?
- How do you cope with everyday living?

2 Learning to live with it - the intermediate stage

This stage is characterized by feelings of disconnectedness and alienation from the family. Some patients emerge from this stage with the knowledge that some strategies reduce their symptoms. These patients feel better able to cope than their counterparts when unfavourable situations arise.

Assessment questions:
- How do you try to control your pain?
- What would you do if you had a flare?
- How often should you exercise?

3 Mastery - final stage

The patient emerges from this stage with a positive perspective about their condition, having acquired knowledge about the disease and how to live with it.

Assessment questions:
- How do you feel about your arthritis?
- Do you feel in charge of it?

Source: Shaul (1995); Ryan (1998)

---

forms. The first occurred when joint tenderness was at its peak and the second when tenderness was reduced. The latter type of depression is the most problematic, as it appears to have a less favourable outcome. Patients in this category can be identified by scrutiny of sequential assessments. Patients whose depression appears to be associated with pain can usually be helped by discussion of pain relief methods (see Table 4.4), but those that do not respond to these therapies or other nursing interventions require a medical referral.

Disability

Psychological factors appear to play an important role in a patient's ability to adapt to their condition (Oberai and Kirwan, 1988), and evidence is accumulating of an association between psychological factors and disability. The importance of this cannot be overestimated, as psychological effects appear to be more accurate at predicting ensuing disability than conventional measures of disease activity (McFarlane and Brooks, 1988).

Both anxiety and depression are common problems and it is important to assess the patient for their presence. The Hospital Anxiety and Depression scale has been devised specifically for use in clinics on patients who do not have a psychiatric diagnosis (Zigmond and Snaith, 1983). It is quick and easy to complete and has predetermined levels indicating the presence of anxiety and depression.

Social effects

Patients with rheumatic diseases may experience social effects, including:

- job loss
- reduced income
- role changes
- relationship changes
- loss of self-esteem
- social exclusion
- transportation problems
- isolation.

Any one of these can have important secondary effects. It may be impossible for a patient to retain their job either outside or inside the home. This can have a financial and psychological impact, as income is lost and self-esteem is affected. Role changes may ensue and valued activities become impossible, resulting in social isolation, often accompanied by depression (Yelin and Callahan, 1995). If these problems are present, it is important that they are detected and addressed. The nurse can give general advice regarding the availability of state assistance, but should also feel able to refer patients to a social worker, Citizens Advice Bureau, disability officer or an agency such as Arthritis Care.

Effects on the family

Family life can be disrupted when chronic disease strikes one of its members and it has been suggested that the impact produces one of three results (Affleck et al., 1988):

- There is minimal alteration in role responsibilities or division of labour.
- There is a positive impact and the family is brought closer together.
- There is a negative impact and the family is driven apart.

Each family is a dynamic social unit and the way in which it adjusts to chronic disease has a significant influence on the outcome for the patient. If the family is understanding and supportive, the patient is more likely to adhere to their treatment regimens (Radojenic et al, 1992; Ryan, 1996b). It is therefore useful for a family member to accompany the patient to the clinic, so that an assessment of family dynamics can be undertaken. If this is not possible, the patient should be encouraged to talk about their situation and how the family members view their disease.

Sexual relationships

Sexuality is an important part of many people's lives and if it is likely that a disease will give rise to problems then it merits investigation. Many nurses feel uneasy about discussing sexuality, which is unfortunate, since patients cite the nurse as the person they would feel most able to approach if they had sexual/relationship problems (Ryan et al., 1996b; Hill et al., 2003b). This places an onus on the professional nurse to at least approach the topic, even if they subsequently refer the patient on to a specialist service such as Sexual Problems Of the Disabled (SPOD).

Painful, disfigured joints, changes to the patient's image of themselves and symptoms such as joint stiffness and fatigue can all have a negative affect on sexual relationships (Hill et al., 2003b). Sexual intercourse can become difficult, as the patient and partner have to contend not only with the symptoms but also with a limited range of joint movement. Some of these problems can be alleviated by sympathetic use of analgesia, warm baths/showers and positional changes. However, some problems, such as erectile dysfunction, are outside the competence of most nurses and will need to be referred to a specialist.

Sexuality has a much broader meaning than the mere act of sexual intercourse. It is an expression of the individual's self-identity and is an integral part of being human (Prady et al., 1998). Relationships are affected and chronic rheumatic diseases can put a strain on both the patient and the healthy partner. Research to date suggests that problems occur more frequently when disease presents in an established relationship (Le Gallez, 1993).

Assessment of these potentially embarrassing problems can be undertaken by use of a questionnaire such as that used in previous research (Hill et al., 2003b).

Patient education

Patient education is an essential element of the role of the rheumatology nurse and plays a central part in enabling patients to manage their own disease. This is important because the majority of patients with severe rheumatic disease are never hospitalized because of their illness, but are managed by a combination of outpatient and GP care. Consequently, effective management depends on the patient's willingness and ability to adhere to their therapies. Patient education is the process by which patients are prepared for this important undertaking (Hill, 1995).

What is patient education?

The provision of information is an important aspect of care, but it is only part of the process we call patient education. Patient education has been defined as:

> any set of planned, educational activities designed to improve patients' health behaviours and/or health status (Lorig, 1996).

The objective of patient education is to bring about behavioural changes that will facilitate improved health status. The chances of success are increased when patient education is underpinned by a proven theory such as self-efficacy theory (Bandura, 1977). Self-efficacy is 'a person's confidence in their ability to perform a specific task or achieve a particular objective'. Those patients who exhibit a high degree of self-efficacy believe that their actions can make a positive difference to their health, and this has an influence on health behaviour and outcomes. Patients who undertake a patient education programme have been shown to develop the positive coping mechanisms necessary to achieve an acceptable quality of life, despite their problems and disabilities (Hill, 2003c).

Patient education can be taught in a number of formats including:

- individual education
- group education
- arthritis self-management programme (a form of group education)
- opportunity education.

All of these formats are discussed in detail in other texts (Hill, 1999). The format most relevant to nurse-led clinics is individual patient education. It is flexible and can be tailored to the specific patient needs, and it allows inclusion of topics that are important to the individual patient (Table 4.6). It also enables the pace and order to be dictated by the patient.

Is patient education effective?

There is abundant evidence of the effectiveness of patient education

Table 4.6 Topics included in a patient education programme

- Knowledge of disease: aetiology, disease process and tests
- Symptom management: non-pharmacological interventions pain, stiffness, fatigue
- Drug treatments: categories of drugs, how to use them effectively, side effects
- Protecting joints: splinting and changing lifestyles
- Exercising: how, what, when
- Diet: reducing/increasing weight, effects on health, fatigue
- Sexual life: sexual activity, contraception, pregnancy
- Coping strategies: contracting, heightening self-efficacy
- Communicating: getting the most out of consultations
- Goal setting: setting achievable targets and reaching them

(Hirano et al., 1994; Hawley, 1995; Hill et al, 2001), and there is concordance in identifying improvements in pain, tenderness, tender joint counts and functional ability. However, the most recent evidence is a Cochrane Review specific to RA (Reimsma et al., 2002). In this work, patient education was shown to have a small but significant effect on anxiety and depression, joint counts, disability and the patient's overall assessment of their condition. Improvements persisted for 3 months, but by 12 months they had disappeared. Of the three forms of intervention scrutinized (counselling, providing information and behavioural treatments), only the last demonstrates significant improvement. Although these results are interesting, no account is taken of the appropriateness of different interventions at different stages of the patient's adjustment to their disease and, as we know, different patients react differently. It is incumbent on the nurse to provide patient education at the right time and at the right speed. Patients may need time to come to terms with their situation, and at this stage the nurse's role is to support and counsel. Providing information can commence when the patient starts seeking information and motivational interviewing will prepare the patient to undertake behavioural changes to their lifestyles. Once the patient is receptive, patient education can commence.

Conclusion

Nurse-led clinics have proven value in the form of greater symptom control and enhanced patient self-care, and as a consequence they are becoming more widespread. This trend is likely to accelerate in response to the more generalized use of new therapies, such as the biologics, which will necessitate the expansion of nurse-led clinics.

This chapter is intended to assist this process by providing guidance to nurses who are new to the speciality and wish to establish a nurse-led clinic. However, rheumatology nursing is a complex activity and the nursing care outlined is simply an overview. For more in-depth knowledge referral to other texts will be necessary.

Chapter 5

Nurse clinics: using the right tools for the job

Sarah Hewlett

Introduction

Until the late 1970s, measuring outcomes in rheumatology was rare. What was being measured was the *process* of disease – inflammatory indices such as erythrocyte sedimentation rate (ESR) and bony damage on x-rays – issues important to the doctor for decision making. However, as our clinical experience tells us, process does not always relate well to outcome, for example the amount of bony damage that a patient experiences in joints does not always indicate difficulty using those joints. A pivotal change took place in 1980 with the publication of the first patient-centred outcome measures (Health Assessment Questionnaire: Fries et al., 1980; Arthritis Impact Measurement Scales: Meenan et al., 1980). These were outcomes thought to be important to patients in their everyday lives. Over the past 20 years the number of available measures has increased dramatically. The wealth of options available means that some clinical professionals may value guidance on the selection process, especially if they are to make best use of the tools available – and particularly if clinical or service decisions are to be made on the basis of such assessments.

At the same time as this surge in production of clinical outcome measures, nursing practice has been developing to a more specialized level with the establishment of nurse-led clinics. Professionally, we are accountable for our practice (Nursing and Midwifery Council, 2002b) and should evaluate our effectiveness in patient care and our use of resources (DoH, 1999c).

This chapter provides practical step-by-step advice on measuring outcomes appropriately in your own nurse-led clinics (see summary of the process in Table 5.1), and is divided into six sections:

- How to select the right outcomes to measure.
- What types of tool are available?

- What are the practical considerations?
- How to ensure the tool is valid
- What are common tools in use?
- Using the results constructively.

The chapter does not attempt to review all known rheumatology outcome measures (a Herculean task) as these can be found elsewhere (Bellamy 1993; Bowling 1997, 2001). Instead, it provides practical guidance for setting up outcome measurement (Figure 5.1).

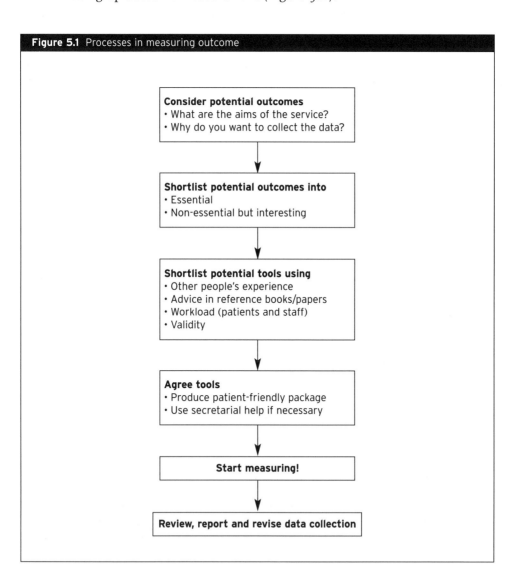

Figure 5.1 Processes in measuring outcome

How to select the right outcomes to measure

Which outcomes might be changed as a result of the intervention?

To decide which outcomes to measure, first consider what the purpose of the nurse-led clinic or service is, and therefore what outcomes it might be appropriate to measure. For example, if the aim of the clinic is to support patients newly diagnosed with rheumatoid arthritis (RA), then a tool to measure knowledge and a tool to measure anxiety might be used in addition to measures of inflammation or disease activity. However, if the aim of the clinic is to educate patients with osteoporosis in the prevention of falls and fractures, then tools to measure posture, balance and diet would be appropriate. Nurse-led clinics can be established for a variety of purposes, including supporting patients with new diagnoses, long-term management of RA, monitoring of second-line therapy, giving biologic agents, self-management, patient education, individual disease clinics (e.g. osteoporosis, connective tissue diseases), rapid access and others. Different clinics with different aims require their own particular set of outcome tools – there is little point in measuring something that a particular clinic or service is not designed to affect. Therefore, if it does not already exist in a clinic protocol, a statement of the prime aim of the clinic should be agreed.

The nurse and multidisciplinary team can then consider which patient outcomes they think will be affected and what sort of changes they think will occur, such as reduction in pain or increase in quality of life (Table 5.1). The nurse should review current and pivotal papers and books on rheumatology nurse-led clinics to get an idea of the sort of outcomes that could be measured (Felson et al., 1993; Hill et al., 1994, 1998; Le Gallez, 1998; RCN, 2001). However, as the patient is often receiving simultaneous care from other colleagues within the multidisciplinary team, it may be that in some cases it is a 'total package' that is being evaluated, rather than a purely nurse-led intervention. A short list of potential outcomes to be measured should be agreed, and divided into 'essential' and 'non-essential but interesting' outcomes.

What is the patient population?

It is important to clarify the patient population, as different diseases have varying consequences for the patient and hence need different outcome tools. For example, the nurse might wish to measure skin involvement in a connective disease clinic, but would not wish to measure this in an RA clinic.

Table 5.1 Some suggestions for outcomes from nurse clinics in rheumatoid arthritis

Inflammatory activity	Function and related concepts
• Pain	• Function or activities of daily living
• Swollen joints	• Mobility
• Tender joints	• Self-care
	• Impact of disability

Mood	Beliefs
• Depression	• Coping
• Anxiety	• Empowerment
• Helplessness	• Self-efficacy
• Anger	• Self-esteem
	• Acceptance of illness
	• Social support
	• Relationships
	• Perceived stress
	• Body image

Self-management	Other issues
• Behaviour change	• Fatigue
• Joint protection	• Sleep
• Exercises	• Skin integrity
• Lifestyle change	• Nutrition/weight
• Adherence to therapy	• Side effects of drugs
• Participation in care	• Use of resources
• Knowledge or understanding	• Satisfaction

Should services issues be measured?

A nurse-led clinic is not a free resource! This is usually obvious when it is being set up as a new service, or additional nurses are needed to expand a service. However, even if the clinic has been long established, there is still value in assessing its cost-effectiveness. Nurse clinics can be assessed for costs incurred (amount of nursing time, number of patients seen, number of referrals made to other team members), costs saved (e.g. effect on waiting lists) and effectiveness (change in patient outcome, patient problems identified and rectified). In addition, satisfaction with the service might be measured.

What is the purpose of collecting the data?

It may be necessary to monitor the patient's condition (e.g. to see if therapies are effective), and these data would be used for individual patient management or clinical care.

The nurse may also wish to collect the data to audit the service provided. Audit is a systematic approach to reviewing care to see if standards are being met and it may identify development opportunities. It does not cause disturbance to the patient beyond normal clinical care. The hospital's audit department is a useful resource for discussing needs. They may have the ability to enter or analyse audit data, or even collect non-clinical data (e.g. waiting times).

Research is a systematic investigation intending to add to knowledge, and it may involve disturbance over and above normal clinical care. Research studies will allow the nurse to calculate statistical differences between or within patients to provide robust evidence in support (or otherwise) of a predetermined hypothesis. For example, a patient may improve following a self-management programme led by a nurse, but it would not be possible to be certain that this improvement was due to the programme unless other treatments (e.g. medication change) had been controlled during the programme. Therefore not only must research studies have a stated hypothesis to test and a strict design to exclude confounding factors, they must also have sufficient numbers to test for a statistically significant answer and to ensure that an effect is not missed (if it is there). Research study design is outside the scope of this chapter and readers are advised to consult a research textbook (e.g. Polgar and Thomas, 1998), experienced researchers or their hospital's research and development department. Research needs to be properly designed, funded and approved in ethics, and comply with research governance requirements (see www.info.doh.gov.uk).

The nurse should also consider who has asked for the data and why. Is it the nurses' decision to measure the efficacy of their clinics? Is it a medical or managerial request? Each group may have a different agenda, such as improving practice, assessing need or assessing cost. Such issues should be fully discussed before deciding on outcomes to be measured to ensure that the nurses are satisfied that there is good reason for the extra effort involved in data collection.

What types of tool are available?

Outcomes can be measured in a variety of ways, but the aim is to obtain maximum accuracy.

Subjective and objective assessment tools

Subjective assessments are reports by the patient of their own health status, often in the form of questionnaires or visual analogue scales (VAS; described in more detail later in this chapter). Objective assessments are those made by an external assessor (e.g. nurse, doctor, other health professional) and can include measures such as laboratory tests (e.g. haemoglobin). Assessments may be made using questionnaires, observing performance (e.g. walking time), by physical examination (e.g. articular index) or by interview (e.g. to assess whether or not the patient is depressed).

It used to be felt that patient self-reports might be influenced by mood, for example a depressed patient might report greater disability because of their overall outlook. However, there is little evidence for this, and it is now generally accepted that patient self-report and objective clinician assessment can provide different views of the same concept and can usefully be used in combination to give a better picture of patient status.

Disease-specific and generic assessment tools

Assessment tools can be specific to a disease or generic (i.e. valid across a range of different diseases such as multiple sclerosis, arthritis, diabetes). Disease-specific questionnaires have an advantage in that they address issues that may be very important in a specific disease (e.g. skin involvement in systemic sclerosis), or components to a particular issue that are very specific (e.g. a generic fatigue measure may not pick up the particular type of fatigue experienced by RA patients). Conversely, generic questionnaires have the advantage that they allow comparison across diseases. For example, if a manager wishes to compare the efficacy of nurse-led clinics in diabetes with those in RA, then they might measure health status in both populations using the SF-36 (Ware and Sherbourne, 1992), which is a generic tool. The nurse should consider what the data is going to be used for before deciding on disease-specific tools, generic tools or both.

Single-topic and multidimensional tools

Questionnaires can either measure a single concept or multiple concepts. Multidimensional tools may give a global score or be broken down into subscales, or both. Some multidimensional questionnaires offer an attractive and comprehensive package of assessment, but the number of items per scale can actually be very few, such that very little data are being used to assess the concept. For example, a multidimensional health status tool might incorporate only two or three items on a depression subscale, compared to a 20-item specific depression scale, which might mean depression is inadequately captured. However, offering patients a large package of single-topic questionnaires that address each concept in great depth can reduce the rate of returned questionnaires (see below).

What are the practical considerations?

Having decided on the outcome to use, it is worth discussing with colleagues, both locally and in the wider forum, what tools are available to measure it. They may have experience of a variety of tools and offer valuable recommendations (or suggest tools to avoid!). Check the books and papers that led to the selection of the nursing outcomes and see which tools they used and whether they might be applicable in the identified area. Try to manage with the smallest number of tools possible, although you may need to use a number if you are measuring several different concepts. Check the sorts of tool available in a reliable assessment reference book that provides overviews of scales to help narrow the field (Bellamy, 1993; Bowling, 1997, 2001). Create a short list of potential tools.

How to locate the potential questionnaires and tools

Start with the validation paper. Find the reference in the papers or books already reviewed. If this proves difficult you will need to do a search for the key papers on the computer (see Appendix 2 for information on useful search facilities). The hospital research and development support unit should have literature-searching facilities and be able to offer you support for this, as may the hospital librarian. To obtain a copy of the paper itself, use the same sources (many hospitals or universities have paid for access to electronic journals via the web), or try the Royal College of Nursing library (see website list) or the local university library, or check with colleagues who may have the journal on their shelves.

How to decide which of the outcome tools to use

Once you have the validation paper, you can review the chosen tool to see if it has been validated satisfactorily (see p. 93). Consider whether the tool proposed is validated in the relevant patient population, e.g. a pain tool validated for osteoarthritis would not necessarily apply to RA patients because of the different nature of the pain in RA. Consider convenience for patient and staff. Again, refer to the reference books for a balanced summary of the scale and its validation, scoring and any important considerations (Bellamy, 1993; Bowling, 1997, 2001).

You will need to check whether the questionnaire or tool is under copyright. Many tools are freely available for use, including their exact wording and scoring mechanisms, having been published in the public domain. However, you may need to purchase the right to use the tool. There is no definitive list of which tools are under copyright, but check first on the nferNelson website (www.nfer-nelson.co.uk), as they hold the copyright for many tools. If the tool chosen is not listed there, search to see if the tool itself has a website created by its authors (e.g. SF-36 website, www.sf-36.org/copyright.shtml). If there is a website, it will state whether or not there is a need to pay to use the tool. If both these searches fail, then it is probably reasonable to assume there is no copyright and the tool can be used. It may be worth looking for a website for the questionnaire in any case, as they often give helpful information or normative data.

Be wary of using measures that have been validated in a different disease population or culture, unless they have also been revalidated in UK populations. If no validated measure exists, do not just draw up a set of questions and assume they measure what they appear to measure (see p. 93). The most defensible action in the absence of a validated questionnaire would probably be to design a simple VAS. But first, take advice from senior nurses or researchers within the national or international rheumatology community on the best way forward.

How much patient effort is involved?

There is a need to balance getting adequately detailed information from long or multiple questionnaires against using as few questionnaires as possible to reduce 'questionnaire fatigue' in patients. Some questionnaires have been produced in shorter formats, which researchers believe still provide equivalent data (e.g. Modified HAQ: Pincus et al., 1983), although authors of the original scales may dispute such claims! Questionnaire fatigue may mean that patients don't complete the whole package, only complete it on some occasions or decline right from the start. However, using shorter packages may reduce the accuracy of the assessment.

If there is a long list of outcomes, capture the essential outcomes first and then discuss whether there is room for those outcomes that are interesting but not essential. If there are several candidate tools for one outcome, then decide which tool is the most appropriate; here the length of the total questionnaire package might be one of the deciding factors, along with validity. Use secretarial support to produce a clean, smart version, where questions are laid out well and aligned properly. Using a faxed questionnaire sample, which has been cut, pasted and then photocopied, is not going to inspire co-operation in your patients! Be honest about how long the questionnaire will take to complete and what it will be used for. In general, patients seem to find questionnaires interesting – within the limits of their ease of completion and perceived usefulness. Finally, to maximize co-operation and reduce questionnaire fatigue, produce the package in a user-friendly format. Many trusts have a patient review group who review all literature for clarity and simplicity of purpose before patients are requested to read or fill in new forms

Patients should be invited to complete the questionnaires and given an explanation as to what they will be used for. They should be told why some questions appear similar and advised that, in general, it is best to enter their first thoughts rather than deliberate over their answers. They should be reassured that their answers will remain confidential. What seems a perfectly reasonable assessment to the nurse may cause concern or confusion for patients, e.g. many articular indices do not examine the feet because of poor reproducibility, yet this may be the patient's most pressing problem. The nurse needs to give a brief explanation and then return to examine the feet for clinical reasons, after the formalized assessment. Such considerations are likely to enhance adherence for questionnaires and assessments.

How much staff workload is involved?

Measuring outcome also takes staff time and effort, as staff must distribute and score the questionnaires, enter and analyse the data, and produce a report. Therefore the nurse should be quite clear about the purpose of measuring outcomes and establish which are core outcomes and which should be measured out of interest only if time and money permit.

The timing of outcome measurements depends on when each individual outcome is expected to respond to the nurses' intervention. How often and for how long the data are collected also depends on this, and on the reason for collecting the data. If the data are being collected for clinical management purposes, then they might be collected at each visit. However, if the data are to examine the efficacy of a specific intervention (e.g. patient self-management programme), then there might be a finite cut-off point for data collection beyond which it would not be expected to see further improvement.

Other tasks to be considered are who is going to score and enter the data, and who is going to review the results. Scoring and data entry could be an administrative rather than a nursing task, but the nurse will want to review the individual and collective results. If the data are entered only in the patient's notes, this makes it difficult to collate them if there is a need to look at collective outcomes, so data might also be entered on a central database. There should be no need to remind either the nurse or the person dealing with the data of the confidentiality of the results.

How to ensure that the tool is valid

It is essential to be as sure as possible that the selected tool measures what it says it does. For example, depression can also manifest itself in physical symptoms such as fatigue; thus a depression questionnaire that contains questions on fatigue might confuse a flare with depression in RA patients. The purpose of this section is not to instruct the reader in questionnaire design – for some researchers this is a full-time job and a questionnaire can take years to develop and validate – but to give guidance on how validation is tackled. This will enable you to assess whether or not the published questionnaire selected has reasonable provenance (Table 5.2).

Table 5.2 Types of validation for an assessment tool

Content validity	Is it comprehensive?
Face validity	Is it credible?
Criterion validity	Is it consistent and accurate?
Discriminant validity	Is it sensitive to change?
Construct validity	Does it make biological sense?

Does it cover all relevant aspects?

Initially, a tool should be developed in a way that ensures that it covers all the relevant aspects of the concept (content validity or comprehensiveness) and that it seems sensible to professionals and patients (face validity or credibility). These two might be covered by the researcher gathering ideas for questions (on say, fatigue) from both patients and professionals, to ensure that the questions reflect the range of experiences of fatigue in arthritis and do not miss out key issues.

Is it consistent and accurate?

Once the issues have been generated and the questions created and collated during development, the tool must tested. First, it is necessary to ensure that it is consistently accurate (criterion validity). This is usually undertaken by testing the new questionnaire twice, in the same group of patients, over a short period, say one week apart. It should be at a time when consistent answers might be expected. In addition, the new scale is usually compared to the best available 'gold standard' completed under the same conditions to assess its accuracy (e.g. compare a new disability scale to the best existing disability questionnaire or an objective measure of observed performance).

Does it detect changes in the patient's condition?

Having made sure that the tool is consistent and accurate, it needs to be assessed for sensitivity to change, that is to see if the questionnaire reflects changes in the patient's condition (discriminant validity). To examine this the researcher might test the questionnaire in patients undergoing a specific intervention that would be expected to change their condition (e.g. a relaxation programme in fatigue), and measure their status before and after the intervention.

Do the results make biological sense?

Finally, the new tool has to be assessed to see if it makes biological sense when compared to other constructs (construct validity). For example, if a new depression scale was not related to anxiety then there would be concerns about its validity, as all the published evidence shows strong associations between anxiety and depression. To test for construct validity the patient could be asked to complete both the new tool and measures of other constructs we would expect to be related. We can then see if the expected associations are present, and also whether any new associations revealed by the data make biological sense. For example, a new fatigue questionnaire might be expected to show that increased fatigue correlates with high inflammatory indices, but, if high fatigue were strongly associated with feelings of wellbeing, it would be difficult to find a sensible biological construct to explain this.

There are many good reference texts on validation of new scales and the five validation issues highlighted above are common to most texts, although some use slightly different labels, leading to potential confusion.

It is a good idea to stick to one text and always use that as a basis for assessing the principles of validation to use on scales; Tugwell and Bombardier (1982) provide a useful framework.

What are common tools in use?

Tools in RA

Providing a detailed description of every scale and its validation would be the subject of a whole book rather than a chapter, and Table 5.3 lists some reliable reference books that give useful descriptions. This section describes some of the most commonly used assessment tools.

Table 5.3 Useful departmental reference textbook

Deciding on nursing outcomes to measure

- Hill J (ed.) (1998) Rheumatology Nursing: a creative approach. Edinburgh: Churchill Livingstone.
- Le Gallez P (ed.) (1998) Rheumatology for Nurses: patient care. London: Whurr.
- Royal College of Nursing (2001) Standards for Effective Practice and Audit in Rheumatology Nursing. London: RCN.

Deciding on specific outcome tools to use

- Bellamy N (1993) Musculoskeletal Clinical Metrology. Lancaster: Kluwer Academic Publishers.
- Bowling A (1997) Measuring Health: a review of quality of life measurement scales, 2nd edn. Buckingham: Open University Press.
- Bowling A (2001) Measuring Disease: a review of disease-specific quality of life measurement scales, 2nd edn. Buckingham: Open University Press.

Inflammatory activity

Pain can be measured in a reliable manner using a pain VAS, which provides a robust measure. A VAS normally comprises a 10 cm horizontal line with a marker and descriptor at each end, descriptors being the extreme ends of the concept being measured (e.g. no pain – severe pain) (Figure 5.2). Patients make a mark on the VAS according to the strength of their problem or belief, and the distance from the initial marker is measured. When reviewing VAS scores, note the direction of the scoring system (e.g. high scores giving worse status) and whether any have been worded in the opposite direction. The horizontal VAS with end markers and end descriptors is a well-validated methodology, but caution should be used if the proposed VAS has additional markers, words or numbers along its length, as these may reduce a 10 cm (100 mm) continuous scale to a 10-item or category scale. Caution should also be used when photocopying from a copy rather than an original, as photocopying can distort the length of the line (Huskisson, 1982). Pain diaries can also be used, where the patient records a pain score regularly (e.g. daily) in the form of a number or category (e.g. 1–4, or none–mild moderate–severe). However, some patients complete these retrospectively while waiting for their appointment, and others report they do not like to be reminded of their pain by such frequent assessments. Recording analgesic use may be helpful, but some patients do not take analgesics even in the face of strong pain, either because they do not feel they work or because of a dislike of tablets. Early morning stiffness is frequently recorded, but the accuracy and reproducibility of this measure are poor (Hazes et al., 1994). Articular indices are a reliable and better way of assessing inflammatory activity, and many have been developed over the years, using different combinations of joints, symptoms and scoring systems. One of the most reliable and frequently used is the 28-joint count (Fuchs et al., 1989), which assesses shoulders, elbows, wrists, metacarpophalangeal joints (MCPs), proximal interphalangeals (PIPs) and knees. Tenderness and swelling are recorded separately (present/absent) and positive joints totalled for each symptom (0–28). This count is quick, reproducible and correlates with serum markers of inflammation. A useful additional measure of inflammatory activity is patient global assessment of how well they are doing (VAS, very well to very badly), alongside a similar physician global assessment. These are included in the seven core outcomes for measuring inflammatory activity recommended by the American College of Rheumatology (tender joints, painful joints, patient assessment of pain, patient global assessment, physician global assessment, function and an acute phase-reactant) (Felson et al., 1993).

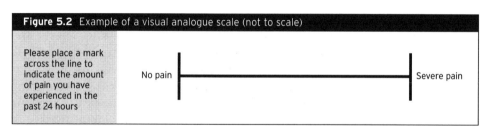

Figure 5.2 Example of a visual analogue scale (not to scale)

Please place a mark across the line to indicate the amount of pain you have experienced in the past 24 hours

No pain |———————————————| Severe pain

Function

The Health Assessment Questionnaire (HAQ: Fries et al., 1980) is a 20-item scale looking at activities of daily living, which has been validated for use in the UK (Kirwan and Reeback, 1986). The questions are divided into eight categories (dress, rise, eat, walk, hygiene, reach, grip and leisure) and questions are answered as 'no difficulty', 'some difficulty', 'much difficulty' or 'unable to do' (score 0–3). There is space for patients to tick aids or assistance that relate to the each of the eight categories. The highest score for each of the eight categories is used and, if the patient has indicated using an aid or assistance in a category that has only scored 0–1, then that score is raised to 2. The eight category scores are totalled (0–24) and then divided by 8 to reach a final average category score of 0–3. This scale is widely used and respected, translated and validated in many cultures, and is probably the gold standard of functional measurement in arthritis. While the HAQ measures function well, it does not measure whether or not these functional difficulties matter to the patient. This 'personal impact' can be measured taking individual values as weights, either by questionnaire (Personal Impact HAQ: Hewlett et al., 2002) or interview (McMaster–Toronto Arthritis Patient Function Preference Questionnaire, McTAR: Tugwell et al., 1990). Other methods of measuring function include performance measures, such as grip strength, the button test or a timed walk. All of these outcomes can vary from day to day, depending on the effort expended, motivation and technique (e.g. footwear in a walking test), and the exuberance of the assessor's encouragement! They take greater time as they require the patient and assessor to be present.

Mood

Anxiety and depression can be measured using the Hospital Anxiety and Depression scale (Zigmond and Snaith, 1983). This 14-item scale has seven questions each for anxiety and depression. Each answer is scored from 0 to 3, giving a total of 0–21 for each scale. This particular scale is useful in RA because, unlike other depression scales, it omits somatic questions that reflect depression but might also reflect physical signs of a flare in RA (e.g. increased pain or tiredness). A score of 7 or less indicates no problem, 8–10 a potential problem, and 11 or above that the patient might benefit from treatment. The scale was designed for general rather than psychiatric outpatients, and is intended as a screening tool. Copyright can be purchased from nferNelson (see www.nfer-nelson.co.uk). In addition, many patients develop feelings of learned helplessness in the face of unpredictable, uncontrollable chronic disease. This concept can be measured using the Arthritis Helplessness Index

(AHI) (Stein et al., 1988). This five-item questionnaire was developed from the original AHI (Nicassio et al., 1985) and uses six categories (strongly agree to strongly disagree). Scores are totalled to give a range from 5 to 30, with higher scores reflecting higher helplessness.

Beliefs

Probably the most common belief to be measured in RA is self-efficacy, or the belief that there is something that individuals can do to make a difference to their condition (Bandura, 1977), and many self-management programmes try to prompt behaviour change by enhancing self-efficacy. The Arthritis Self-Efficacy scale (ASES) (Lorig et al., 1989) has subscales for pain, function and other symptoms, although the function subscale is less commonly used as experience shows it to be apparently less sensitive to change. The three subscales have five, nine and six VAS questions respectively, and for each subscale the scores are totalled and averaged, with high scores indicating high self-efficacy. The ASES was developed in the USA and is widely used. An RA-specific scale has been developed in the UK (Rheumatoid Arthritis Self-Efficacy scale: Hewlett et al., 2001), for which sensitivity to change is currently being tested. Perceived stress and methods of coping are complex issues to measure and the reader is directed elsewhere for more detailed advice (Bowling, 2001).

Quality of life

The Disease Repercussion Profile (Carr, 1996) comprises six areas of life affected by arthritis that were raised as important by RA patients (function, social activities, relationships, emotions, socio-economic issues and body image). Patients are asked to rate how important the effect of arthritis is in each of these areas (0–10) and to enter free text about these problems, making it a potentially useful tool in clinic discussions. The copyrighted tool is available from Alison Carr (Rheumatology Department, the University of Nottingham). The RA Quality of Life scale (RAQoL: De Jong et al., 1997) uses 30 items, also derived from patients, with yes/no answers, giving a range of 0–30, with a higher score indicating a poorer quality of life. This straightforward scale is available from Galen Research (galen@galen-research.com).

Multidimensional scales

The Arthritis Impact Measurement scales (AIMS-2: Meenan et al., 1992) uses 78 items arranged in 12 subscales, measuring function, social life, pain, work, tension and mood, and also satisfaction and prioritization questions (copyrighted). A useful generic tool is the Short Form 36 (SF-36: Ware and Sherbourne, 1992), which assesses nine health concepts (physical function, physical role, emotional role, social function, pain, mental health, vitality, general health, health transition). Scoring is easiest with a computer-scoring package, which can be obtained with the copyrighted questionnaire (available from www.sf-36.org/copyright.shtml).

Tools used in other types of arthritis

In osteoarthritis, the Western Ontario McMaster Universities Arthritis Index (WOMAC: Bellamy et al., 1988) is a commonly used, robust tool assessing pain, function and stiffness using three subscales with 24 items. Likert scoring is usually used (none, mild, moderate, severe, extreme), although a VAS version exists.

In systemic lupus erythematosus the British Isles Lupus Assessment Group developed the BILAG index (Hay et al., 1993), which assesses eight areas (mucocutaneous, neurological, musculoskeletal, cardiovascular and respiratory, vasculitic, renal, haematological and general). It is complex to score manually, but there is a computer-scoring package available (see www.limathon.com/BLIPS).

In ankylosing spondylitis, pain and stiffness are helpful measures and tragus-to-wall measurement can be useful, as can chest expansion or finger-to-floor distance (a combined policy with the physiotherapy team may be beneficial).

In fibromyalgia, a tender point count may be useful for diagnosis, but, in terms of monitoring outcome, a VAS for fatigue, along with a measure of anxiety and depression, might be appropriate. However, frequent measurement may not be helpful if it serves only to remind patients of their concerns.

In osteoporosis, the measurement of tragus-to-wall distance or dietary reviews may be helpful, and measures could be usefully discussed with physiotherapists if they are providing education on balance and posture.

Using the results constructively

The data may be being collected as part of normal clinical care and used to make clinical decisions in outpatients. Measures of inflammatory activity and function are particularly useful, as the questions or examination of joints can be used as the basis for discussion of problems and potential solutions. The more complex questionnaires of mood, beliefs and quality of life require scoring, but their overall answers can also act as a prompt for further enquiry. The data can be used to show change in the individual patient, which can be documented; some units keep continuous patient records in graph form.

Audit data should be used to examine whether the clinic meets agreed standards on service issues (e.g. response time to helpline calls) and clinical issues (e.g. increase in patient knowledge, reduction in anxiety). The data are a useful indicator of how the nurse, the service and the patients are doing, but be aware that they cannot provide strong statistical evidence for an intervention. It may be necessary to collate audit results and present them to nursing colleagues, the multidisciplinary team or department managers (remember to ensure that patients cannot be identified). This can be valuable in helping to develop or justify the current service, and can be a useful tool for reviewing and altering practice. It can be a useful exercise to collect audit data intermittently (e.g. twice a year for service issues, or annually for clinical care data), as this reduces data collection workload but allows regular monitoring and comparison. The data may provoke further inquiry and possibly lead to the formulation of a research question.

Research data should be used to answer the research question or hypothesis posed. Advice and support can usually be obtained from the research and development support unit at the hospital, or colleagues experienced in research. The findings should ideally be presented not only to local colleagues but also through abstracts submitted to national and international meetings (e.g. RCN Rheumatology Forum, British Health Professionals in Rheumatology, European League Against Rheumatism, American Rheumatology Health Professionals). Finally, the nurse should consider writing up the research for full publication.

The review or report may lead to a reconsideration of the outcomes being measured due to practical difficulties or apparent inappropriateness of the scales. None of us gets it completely right the first time! Retaining a file of the collated information on the outcome tools (e.g. validation papers, relevant papers using the tool, the questionnaire and scoring system) will save time when they are needed for future reference and will be helpful for other staff in the department.

Conclusions

Nursing has generally been overlooked in the setting of national targets. However, this may well change as nursing becomes an increasing focus for government initiatives. There will then be a more pressing need to identify clearly the benefits (or otherwise!) of nursing care and it will become essential to collect data on nursing services and patient outcome. Outcome measurement is therefore a very useful, if not essential, tool for the nurse setting up a rheumatology service. Like everything in life, there are potential pitfalls, but a systematic approach and appropriate selection of tools will aid the nurse and steer projects or new interventions to a successful implementation and conclusion.

Chapter 6

Drug monitoring: primary or secondary care?

Diane Home and Susan Oliver

Introduction

Drug-monitoring clinics are becoming a valuable resource in healthcare, with adverse drug reactions (ADRs) being a major clinical problem, accounting for 2–6% of all hospital admissions (Pirmohamed et al., 1998). The example of rheumatoid arthritis (RA) and the monitoring needs of disease-modifying anti-rheumatic drug (DMARD) therapies provide the overall framework for this chapter. There are many specialities that use some, if not all, the DMARDs outlined here, and the use of clinics to monitor DMARDs for RA is a useful example for other areas of care that prescribe similar therapies (e.g. nephrology, respiratory, gastroenterology and dermatology). The specific drug dosages, monitoring needs and side-effect profiles may vary, depending on the medical condition, but the needs of the patient and responsibilities of the nurse remain similar in most cases.

In 2002, Bandolier identified that ADRs affected in the region of 7% of inpatient admissions. Antibiotics, anticoagulants, digoxin, diuretics, hypoglycaemic agents and non-steroidal anti-inflammatory drugs (NSAIDs) accounted for 60–70% of all ADRs leading to hospital admission or causing an episode while the patient was in hospital. In addition, the National Patient Safety Agency (NPSA) has been set up to promote safety in all aspects of drug administration and to collate national data on drug incidents. The NPSA works with key organizations to co-ordinate NHS reporting of adverse events and 'near misses' in healthcare and support developments that will reduce risk and improve care (NPSA, 2002).

Initially, practitioners used additional guidelines or patient group directions (PGDs) that provided a document enabling nurses and pharmacists to administer some treatments. Although PGDs provided an early opportunity for nurses and pharmacists to supply and administer therapies, they were not intended to be used as an all-encompassing legislative framework to enable prescribing of treatments and altering of drug dosages.

It is essential that nurses managing drug-monitoring clinics or supporting the service are knowledgeable on the drugs prescribed, side-effect profiles and latest evidence in relation to the therapies (Nursing and Midwifery Council, 2002c). Two important issues have supported this need: the Chief Nursing Officer's ten key roles for nurse development (see Appendix 1) and the development of supplementary prescribing for appropriately trained nurses and pharmacists (DoH, 2003a).

It is clear to all nurses providing care to chronic disease patient groups that there has been an increasing need for nurses either to provide drug-monitoring clinics or to support monitoring regimens by providing expert advice. These additional demands stem from advances in pharmacological options, as well as the growing elderly and chronic disease populations. Whatever the reason, these increases have had a significant impact on the numbers of patients requiring drug monitoring and consequently the provision of effective monitoring.

The method of initiating treatment, patient (and family) education and organization of drug monitoring is an integral part of the planning and development of many chronic disease nursing services. Indeed, it is possible that, in the future, the core principles of long-term medical conditions that lend themselves to chronic disease management clinics could include aspects of drug monitoring as well as assessment of disease control. Nurses working in other speciality fields will find these issues relevant to their own areas of interest, although there may be a need to extend or develop the core principles to encompass specific aspects relating to their own specialist area and specific patient needs.

The information provided in this chapter should enable the reader to:

- review the systems or models of drug monitoring that are currently used in the UK
- discuss the role of the nurse in a monitoring clinic
- discuss the evidence for the monitoring of DMARDs
- provide practical help in developing a monitoring service.

It is beyond the remit of this chapter to describe in detail the range of drug treatments discussed.

Drug treatment in rheumatic diseases

Drug treatment with DMARDs forms a significant component of the management of patients with rheumatic diseases. In RA, the aim of treatment should be to suppress both the clinical and laboratory signs of inflammation in order to prevent joint damage and disability from occurring (Maddison, 2001).

Until the end of the 1980s, the treatment approach to RA was referred to as the 'therapeutic pyramid'. Patients were initially treated with 'first-line' therapies, i.e. well-tolerated drugs associated with low toxicity, such as analgesics and NSAIDs. If these proved ineffective, patients were moved up the pyramid to more toxic, 'second-line' treatments. Examples of second-line drugs were anti-malarials, penicillamine and gold salts. Corticosteroids were the next step up the pyramid, followed by cytotoxic agents, which were sometimes referred to as 'third-line' drugs.

However, research evidence highlighted the fact that joint destruction occurs early in the disease, with the greatest rate of damage taking place during the first two to three years (van Leeuwen et al., 1993). Prolonged suppression of inflammation slows or prevents the progression of joint erosions (Stenger et al., 1998) and, ultimately, treating patients early in the course of their disease is likely to reduce functional disability. Therefore, the current management strategy is to treat RA early with DMARDs. Referral guidelines suggest that early and prompt treatment (within 12 weeks from symptom onset) may improve long-term outcomes for the patient (Emery et al., 2002).

This management strategy means that patients are exposed to drugs associated with greater toxicity profiles from the earliest stages of their disease process. For patients, this means that they have to consider the risks versus benefits of the drug before commencing the treatment. In these early stages, patients may perceive that the drug will cause them more problems than those they are currently experiencing as a result of the disease. Therefore, they need information about the medication along with the opportunity and time to discuss their options. For the rheumatology service this presents the challenge of meeting these needs, along with monitoring greater numbers of patients throughout the entire course of their disease. It has been suggested that the provision of this element of care is proving to be one of the most difficult aspects for rheumatology services (Byrne, 1998) because of the organizational infrastructure required and increasing patient numbers.

This chapter will discuss models of drug monitoring and the role of the nurse in monitoring clinics, highlighting evidence-based practice and practical issues related to providing a drug monitoring service.

Why monitor?

There are two main reasons for monitoring DMARD therapy:

- identification of toxicity or ADRs
- assessment of the efficacy of treatment.

In the context of DMARD therapy, the safety aspect of identifying toxicity is the primary reason for drug monitoring. Wolfe (1997) identifies that DMARDs are associated with many potential ADRs, the most severe of which include malignancy, organ failure, opportunistic infection and death. Therefore, in view of these potential risks, most rheumatologists recommend regular blood testing to monitor for the occurrence of ADRs (Comer et al., 1995). The British Society for Rheumatology (BSR) has published guidelines for DMARD monitoring (BSR, 2000). However, although these guidelines provide an overall framework, there is a lack of strong evidence-based research on the optimum frequency for monitoring of DMARD treatments. It is for this reason that frequency of blood monitoring varies depending on locally agreed guidelines.

The regularity of blood and urine testing in patients receiving these treatments provides an opportunity for the second aspect of monitoring, which is to assess the efficacy of the treatment. This may be done through blood testing for inflammatory markers. However, it has recently been proposed that composite scores of disease activity taken on a regular basis (possibly every visit or every 3 months) to assess for inflammation should be part of the management of RA patients (Fransen et al., 2002) in order to:

- Understand if the chosen therapy is needed and effective
- assess that disease activity is under control
- identify and prevent over-treatment
- identify rapidly advancing disease
- support the choice of specific DMARDs
- titrate DMARD doses against disease activity
- support treatment expectations.

Interestingly, in the past few years, an additional reason to measure disease activity has arisen, that is the emergence of biologic therapies. The time and resources to identify patients who are eligible for biologic therapies according to a high disease activity score (DAS > 5.1) have produced additional pressure for nurses. For specific guidance on biologic therapies see Chapter 8.

In many areas, the drug-monitoring clinic is the most accessible area to commence additional assessments (such as the DAS), although the provision of nursing expertise and the increasing workload have caused tensions for many services. The constraints on services are currently confined to rheumatology departments, although biologic therapies are increasingly being introduced to other medical specialities (e.g. respiratory, renal, gastroenterology and dermatology). Nurses should be aware of the needs of potential new therapies when planning the long-term provision of monitoring clinics.

The role of the nurse in a drug-monitoring service

Drug monitoring is one of the core roles of rheumatology specialist nurses. Phelan et al. (1992) found that 86% of nurse specialists in rheumatology carry out drug monitoring. The Arthritis Research Campaign (Carr, 2001) undertook workshops to define core competencies of all allied healthcare professionals, and it was clear from the workshops that the nurse's role in drug management includes a wide range of responsibilities in addition to the task of providing a monitoring clinic. Eighty per cent of nurses routinely provided information and advice to patients (a significant amount of this would include drug information), 72% routinely read and recorded blood results, 54% routinely requested investigations as well as carrying out drug monitoring. For many nurses, this is carried out within the context of a nurse-led clinic, where all aspects of the patient's care are considered (Hill et al., 1994); for others it is in a dedicated drug-monitoring clinic. However the monitoring is organized, ideally the patient should be seen by the same practitioner at every visit to enhance continuity of care.

The nurse's role at the first visit

At the initial visit the nurse should assess the patient's understanding of arthritis, their drug therapy and their expectations of treatment in order to provide appropriate care and education. The value of patient education in increasing patient adherence has been described by Hill and Johnson (2001) and in Chapter 4. DMARDs are often commenced at a time in the disease process when the patient is experiencing high levels of inflammatory activity, leading to increased symptoms of pain, stiffness, fatigue, anxiety and depression; therefore nursing interventions need to take the circumstances of each individual patient into account. It may be helpful for the patient to invite their partner, a family member or friend to attend the appointment to help them with recollection of the consultation. The nurse should ensure that she does all of the following:

- Give a full explanation of the DMARD including:
  - the purpose of the drug and its rationale for use at this time
  - details of the route, dose and administration
  - the monitoring requirements
  - the potential side effects and what to report and how/who to contact
  - the length of time the drug will take to become effective.
- Provide opportunity to discuss concerns and anxieties.
- Ensure that the appropriate screening tests have been carried out, e.g. liver function tests in the case of methotrexate.
- Discuss any issues specific to the DMARD being commenced, e.g. fertility and contraception issues with methotrexate or leflunomide.
- Provide the patient with a written information sheet about the drug (see useful addresses in Appendix 3) and a patient-held monitoring record book.
- Plan monitoring follow-up appointments.

The nurse's role at follow-up visits

At follow-up visits, the nurse's role is to assess the safety of the patient through clinical and laboratory measures.

The nurse should:

- Assess whether the patient is taking the correct dose in the correct way, e.g. ensuring that methotrexate is being taken weekly.
- Ensure that the patient is taking additional treatments where appropriate, e.g. combination therapy or folic acid co-prescribed with methotrexate.
- Monitor to ascertain if any drug reactions have occurred (Table 6.1).
- Review other prescriptions (e.g. NSAIDs) that may be having an adverse effect on the blood picture or causing side effects.
- Take urine and blood tests according to the monitoring protocol.
- Review blood results and look for any trends or significant changes in the blood picture that may indicate a need to review or discontinue treatment.
- Explain to the patient the relevance of their blood results and, if the patient wishes, extend their knowledge on drug monitoring and identification of trends.
- Provide advice on management of side effects, e.g. if the patient is experiencing headaches and nausea during the initial stages of sulphasalazine, advise the patient to reduce to a lower dose for a further week prior to re-challenging at higher doses.

Table 6.1 Adverse drug reactions associated with DMARDs

What are we looking for during a monitoring appointment?

Skin	Rashes Unexplained bruising Pruritis
Gastrointestinal system	Mouth ulcers/stomatitis Taste impairment Nausea/Vomiting Anorexia/Weight loss Diarrhoea
Renal system	Haematuria Proteinuria Abnormalities in urea and electrolytes
Haematological	Anaemia (this may be associated with chronic disease particularly if normochromic and normocytic) Thrombocytopenia (unexplained bruising or bleeding) Leucopenia Neutropenia Note: It is important to observe for any downward trend in blood counts as well as abnormal results. A downward trend over three tests, even if the absolute figure is still in the normal range, may indicate an adverse drug reaction and appropriate action should be taken. Equally, a sudden elevation or steady increasing trend in white cell count may indicate an infection
Hepatic system	Elevated liver enzymes (Note: elevated alkaline phosphatase and gamma-glutamyl transferase (GGT) may be associated with increased inflammatory activity). Liver function test results may be abnormal if blood tests are not processed promptly. A repeat blood test may be necessary
Respiratory system	Patients complaining of a troublesome dry cough that presents with or without shortness of breath/breathless should be referred urgently for a medical opinion to exclude drug induced pneumonitis. Note: A cough productive of sputum together with a high white cell count may indicate a chest infection precipitating a flare of disease. A sputum specimen may assist in diagnosis and early treatment of chest infections
Immune system	Increased vulnerability to infections

This table is not exhaustive and therefore does not include toxicities associated with each individual DMARD; readers are advised to review local and national policies and individual drug summary of product characteristics (SPCs).

- Document previous results in the drug-monitoring booklet and monitoring card.
- Provide the opportunity to discuss any concerns or anxieties that the patient may have about their treatment, such as interactions with other medications.
- Monitor for signs of increased disease activity that may indicate that the drug is not controlling the disease adequately.

Models of drug monitoring

This section describes the models of drug monitoring currently practised within the NHS. In many areas of care, a wide range of potentially toxic drugs are prescribed with a limited infrastructure to support regular monitoring and review of treatment. The key aspect of ensuring the provision of detailed patient information on drug treatments, blood monitoring and ongoing support often requires the underpinning of a specialist nursing role. This applies to all models of monitoring, as the key to effective management rests with ample opportunities to communicate and support practitioners caring for patients on DMARDs.

When considering the organization of monitoring, it is important to examine the strengths and weaknesses of each system, the resources that are required and/or available to the service, and any arrangements that are already in place. Particular local issues may also be important, such as whether the trust serves a densely populated urban area or a widely spread rural population.

An audit of UK rheumatologists (Comer et al., 1995) identified that the majority (70%) of monitoring was carried out via shared care arrangements between the rheumatologist and GP. Forty per cent were described as ad hoc, while 30% were formalized through the use of guidelines. Of the remainder, 10% were solely hospital-based systems and 6% were entirely GP-based. With the emergence of clinical governance there has been increasing pressure for all units to ensure that they have recognized frameworks for monitoring patients that have been agreed within their local organization. Indeed, there are national agendas (e.g. National Institute for Clinical Excellence) that support the need to develop regionally or, where possible, nationally agreed guidelines for treatment interventions. The drivers for improvement and change in monitoring have also been supported by documents highlighting the inclusion of the patient as an active participant in their care and the need to improve the patient's experience through their healthcare journey (DoH, 2001b). It is clear from research evidence that concordance and patient satisfaction can be improved by improving the quality of interactions between patient and practitioners (Cameron, 1996; Oliver, 1997).

Over the past few years there has been an increase in the number of clinics that include some aspects of drug monitoring. These include the monitoring of:

- warfarin
- drugs used to treat epilepsy
- drugs used to treat dermatological conditions
- drugs used to treat asthma/chronic obstructive pulmonary disease
- drugs used to treat diabetes
- drugs used to treat osteoporosis.

Drug monitoring in secondary care

In secondary care drug monitoring, the sole responsibility for carrying out blood tests, interpreting and documenting results lies with the hospital. Operational details differ from department to department. For example, patients may attend the hospital for a drug-monitoring appointment with a member of the rheumatology nursing staff on each occasion that they require blood-monitoring tests. Alternatively, the patient may be issued with enough blood forms to have their tests taken by the hospital phlebotomy service between each follow-up appointment.

Strengths of secondary care monitoring

- Direct access to the rheumatology service on a monthly basis.
- Patient-held treatment monitoring cards which encourages patient participation and responsibility.
- Continuity of therapeutic interventions.
- Monitoring by nurses with specialist experience and knowledge of DMARDs.
- Development of a therapeutic relationship between the patient and staff.
- Early identification of patients who fail to attend.

This model provides the patient with frequent access to nursing staff with an understanding of RA and its treatment, thus allowing for timely intervention if the patient has a particular problem or concern about their condition. The nurse can give advice and reassurance about DMARDs, such as the identification and management of side effects, which may prevent unnecessary discontinuation of treatment. As already mentioned, the use of DMARDs is recommended as early as possible in the disease process, and the frequent, ongoing appointments that the patient attends in this model provide an opportunity for regular, individual, patient education about their prescribed DMARD. If the patient misses their appointment, the nurse is able to identify this easily and can follow the patient up to explore what has happened.

Weaknesses of secondary care monitoring

- Increasing patient numbers may overwhelm the service.
- The patient may become dependent on the rheumatology department.
- Patient anxiety may be increased by the perception of numerous hospital visits.
- Patient inconvenience, especially attending during working hours.
- Inappropriate consultations about 'general practice problems'.
- Reliance on one member of staff to run the service.
- Large administration burden.
- Division of roles and responsibilities when DMARDs are prescribed by the GP and monitoring is carried out at the hospital.
- Primary care teams are reliant on secondary care knowledge and expertise.

The main weaknesses associated with setting up this type of service are related to resource issues. Nurses who have experience of RA and DMARD monitoring are required; however, many departments may have only one or possibly two members of nursing staff. Byrne (1998) reports that many rheumatology nurses have been victims of their own success, and have set up single-handed monitoring clinics which are now stretched beyond safety limits. There may also be no formal clerical help allocated to the service, and responsibility can fall on the nursing staff. Indeed, these issues highlight the need to develop a clear business case that includes the necessary infrastructure to support the development before providing a new service (see Chapter 2). As Byrne rightly highlights, the provision of such services often rests on a finite amount of specialist nursing expertise. The lack of nurses with specialist expertise has become an increasing problem in many areas of healthcare and it is an issue that needs to be considered when planning a service provision.

In secondary care monitoring, patients may wait until their hospital appointment before seeking help about a problem with their RA, resulting in a delay to treatment. Alternatively, they may take the opportunity to complain about other medical problems rather than attending their GP surgery. There are increasing numbers of patients taking DMARDs and the potential to overwhelm hospital-based services is high. It is for this reason that alternatives to this model have been developed.

Drug monitoring in primary care

Drug monitoring in primary care is also referred to as 'shared care'. In a report by the British Society of Rheumatology in conjunction with the Royal College of Physicians (1992), it is suggested that monitoring and continued prescribing may be shared between secondary and primary care, but that systems need to be established to prevent failure of individual follow-up. In this model, the clinical care of the patient is shared between primary and secondary care. In some areas, the initiation of treatment and early monitoring may be undertaken at the hospital before the patient is referred to the primary care setting (Helliwell and O'Hara 1995). There are some difficulties with the transfer of patients following initiation of treatment, and it is essential that there are excellent communication channels between primary and secondary care to ensure that an additional risk is not introduced with patient monitoring 'falling between' primary and secondary care.

The GP or more usually the practice nurse undertakes the blood testing and interpretation of results within guidelines or protocols developed by the hospital in conjunction with the GP. This system requires excellent communication between all parties to ensure that the correct monitoring occurs and that a fail-safe mechanism is in place to take action in the event of abnormal results. Access to specialist nursing advice needs to be provided to the primary care team to enhance good communication and allow knowledge and expertise to develop in the primary care setting. This is of particular importance because of the increasing monitoring burden in primary care that leaves the GP overwhelmed and under-resourced, with often only limited knowledge of the specialist field of practice.

As the primary care team become more actively involed in shared-care monitoring they will gain expertise in the overall management of the patient. As this expertise develops, it can help primary care teams to recognize the difference between maintaining effective disease control and other contributing factors that may alter the blood picture (e.g. consecutive drops in platelet numbers from a high level may be an indicator of improved disease control rather than an indicator of drug toxicity). Primary care teams who are less informed may stop treatment unnecessarily due to lack of experience in chronic disease blood monitoring. Although this is the safest route in these circumstances, it does affect the patient's management, as it may then be necessary for them to wait to be reviewed by the rheumatology department before being advised about continuing treatment.

In many areas, the provision of telephone helpline services can provide support for the primary care team when undertaking shared-care monitoring regimens (see Chapter 3).

The model of shared-care monitoring in primary care will vary according to:

- historical links with secondary care (e.g. regular formal education)
- knowledge and expertise of primary care physicians
- resources in primary care (e.g. sufficient phlebotomy services and practice nurse expertise)
- patient population and geographical location (e.g. large rural catchment area makes travelling to hospital a significant burden to patients)
- clinical risk and clinical governance perspective based on expertise and infrastructures to support service (e.g. computer technology to support easy access to laboratory tests)
- easy access to secondary care expertise when guidance is needed.

Strengths of shared-care monitoring

- Ease of patient access – more convenient location and appointment time (e.g. those working).
- Patient-held treatment monitoring cards encourage patient participation and responsibility.
- Helps to change the patients' perceptions of coping with their disease. Hospital care perceived as for the 'sick'.
- Enhances the interrelationship of patient, primary care team and specialist services.
- Provides development opportunities and increased satisfaction for primary care staff.
- Increases primary care teams' awareness of overall specialist management, including risks, benefits and side effects of treatment.
- Cascades knowledge and expertise in specialist management.
- Small numbers in each practice create less of an administrative burden. In a general practice of 2000 there may be 20 patients with RA, of whom five may be on DMARD therapy (Helliwell and O'Hara, 1995).
- Prescribing can be directly linked to monitoring, providing a safety mechanism for identification of patients who are not being monitored.
- Frees time in secondary care for more specialized or complex issues.

Weaknesses of shared-care monitoring

- Lack of infrastructure, such as facilities for phlebotomy and collection of samples.
- Lack of trained healthcare professional contact, e.g. phlebotomist takes bloods but has no contact with the practice nurse or GP.
- Shared-care monitoring cards poorly completed or 'held' by primary care team.

- Lack of specialized knowledge and experience of rheumatology in primary care.
- Small numbers of patients can make it difficult to build up knowledge base.
- Perceived lack of time for primary care colleagues to carry out this additional role.
- Lack of continuity with different staff carrying out monitoring.
- Poor computer technology or expert knowledge to identify trends in the blood picture.
- Limited ability to interpret blood results taking into account changes in disease activity (e.g. consecutive drops in haemaglobin level may indicate active disease rather than being a side effect of treatment).
- There can be doubts about legal prescribing/monitoring responsibilities between primary and secondary.

A number of audits have been carried out to examine the safety, effectiveness and problems of shared-care monitoring. Helliwell and O'Hara (1995) audited the monitoring of 249 patients with RA. They found that in 65% of cases the monitoring complied with the protocol (93% for methotrexate, 67% for sulphasalazine and 26% for sodium aurothiomalate). The reason that the sodium aurothiomalate percentage was so low related to the need to obtain a chest x-ray prior to or during treatment. Protocol failures occurred in 22% of patients and were due to the failure to perform timely blood and urine checks. The authors suggest the following reasons for these results:

- Poor communication among GPs, patients and hospitals.
- Lack of clarity about whose responsibility it was to initiate the drug-monitoring appointment – the patient or the GP.
- Logistical problems with transporting specimens to the laboratory.
- Difficulties with taking blood from patients who required domiciliary visits.

Changes were made to the monitoring systems following the audit, such as the introduction of customized monitoring cards, general practice information packs, a telephone helpline and recording of blood test results on monitoring cards by the pathology staff. When the DMARD monitoring was re-audited in 100 consecutive patients (Helliwell and O'Hara, 1997), the percentage in whom the defined monitoring protocol was followed increased from 65% to 83%. The lack of appropriate blood test was cited as the main reason for protocol failure.

Havelock (1998) audited the shared-care booklets of patients attending a rheumatology outpatient department to ascertain whether the monitoring carried out in primary care complied with the guidelines produced by the hospital. Of the 145 patients questioned, 14 did not own a booklet, while 18 had not brought it to the appointment. A total of 113 booklets were examined, and these revealed that 45% of patients were having the recommended number of full blood counts, 30% were having more than expected and 25% were having fewer. Two per cent of those audited were having no monitoring at all.

Monitoring documentation

Monitoring cards

Monitoring cards are used in secondary care monitoring. They are usually locally developed, although some pharmaceutical companies may supply them for specific drugs. They take the form of a table, which details the date, dose, blood and urine results, along with any additional results specific to that drug, e.g. blood pressure. An example can be seen in Figure 6.1. A column may also be included where comments can be

Figure 6.1 Drug-monitoring card

Name	Phone numbers		Diagnosis		
	H				
Address	W		Treatment	Start	Stop
	M				

Date	Dose	ESR	Hb	WBC	Neutro-phils	Plate-lets	AST	ALP	CRP	Urine Protein	Haem	Comments

Other medications:

added, such as details of the administration of a joint or depomedrone injection or the presence of a concomitant illness, which may have an impact on the blood results. Some departments also document other measures, such as disease activity scores or joint counts.

One of the advantages of using such a system is that the format makes the identification of abnormal results and downward trends straightforward and much less time-consuming than trawling though a patient's notes for previous results. In some circumstances units hold a shared drug monitoring card or database of current medications within the department. This means that when the medical notes are not readily accessible some information is available about the patient's current DMARD treatment and blood results. This can be helpful when patients phone the helpline with queries as it provides an overview of previous treatments, dosages and reason for stopping treatment.

Shared-care monitoring booklets

Shared-care booklets are used to facilitate communication between primary and secondary care in both models of drug monitoring and are recommended in the joint report by the British Society of Rheumatology and the Royal College of Physicians (1992). The booklet is held by the patient and is taken to appointments at the GP surgery and the hospital. Helliwell and O'Hara (1995) found that there was unanimous agreement from GPs that shared-care booklets were helpful, and they identified them as one of the key elements of successful shared-care monitoring. Information documented in the booklet includes the date, dose, and blood and urine test results. These booklets can be obtained from pharmaceutical companies; however, many departments produce their own, which may include contact details, monitoring regimens and patient information about the treatment and its side effects.

Interestingly, patients' views on access to a patient-held, shared-care monitoring booklet have not been fully evaluated. However, initiatives by the Department of Health (2001b) and patient groups have highlighted the need to include the patient in the decision-making process. The use of a shared-care monitoring system should be applauded, particularly if monitoring encourages the active participation of the patient in their care. Although the use of patient-held, shared-care monitoring booklets has not been researched in rheumatology care, it would be interesting to know whether such interventions have a positive effect on patient satisfaction, concordance and reducing risk from adverse events (e.g. patient early identification of sudden or consistent drop in white cell counts).

Frequently asked questions

Who is responsible for doing the monitoring?

The NHS Management Executive (1991) has stated that 'the doctor who has clinical responsibility for a patient should undertake the prescribing'; this has been translated into practice in a number of ways. Helliwell and O'Hara (1995) found that there was disquiet about whose responsibility it was to do the monitoring and prescribing. In their opinion, if the GP is prescribing the DMARD therapy then they should also be performing the monitoring. However, this differs around the country. In some places the complete opposite is happening, with secondary care monitoring and prescribing. In others there is a division between the two: GPs are prescribing but hospitals are monitoring and using shared-care documentation to inform the GPs of the monitoring results.

The argument against secondary care prescribing and monitoring is that it fragments the prescribing for each individual patient. This could become a particular problem with potential interactions, e.g. if the patient was prescribed trimethoprim by the GP but was already taking methotrexate prescribed by the hospital. It would seem that there is no absolute answer to this question, but, whichever system is implemented, all parties need to understand their roles and responsibilities and have clear lines of communication.

What are the legal implications if something goes wrong with monitoring?

As has been discussed, the legal aspects of DMARD monitoring with various models have been difficult to interpret with confidence, as some issues have not been fully tested in a court of law. However, in legal terms, the physician who writes the prescription for the drug is accountable for this prescription. There are difficulties in interpreting this issue too. For instance, if a family doctor has been advised by the consultant rheumatologist to prescribe a specific DMARD under ratified local guidelines (by the trust) it could be argued that they are equally accountable provided they have both adhered to the agreed guidelines. However, this issue, as far as the authors are aware, has not been challenged in a court of law. There are a number of important points to remember:

- Duty of care - as applied to the Bolam test. This is set out in the Code of Professional Conduct (Nursing and Midwifery Council, 2002b).

Table 6.2 Legal issues in drug prescribing and monitoring

Legal aspects of risk	Areas of specific risk
The correct drug *Prendergast v Sam and Dee 1989**	• Clarity of prescription request • Verbal versus written • Competency and authority to request treatment (e.g. various steroids) • **Communication**
The correct dosage *Kay v Ayrshire & Arran HB 1986** *Dwyer v Rodrick 1983**	• How many times per day (e.g. methotrexate weekly)? • Calculated on weight • **Communication**
The correct route/site *Griffin v University Hospital Birmingham NHS Trust, 1998**	• Subcutaneous/intramuscular/ intravenous
Drug interactions	• Knowledge of interactions • Recognition of signs of interactions • Action necessary • **Communication**
The correct withdrawal *Hartwell v South West Metropolitan Regional Health Board 1976**	• Stopping treatment and consequences • Follow-up management • **Communication**
Clarity of responsibility Shared care *Wiltshire v Essex Ara HA 1988**	• Who administers? • Who monitors? • Side-effect strategy • Patient consent/awareness • Team liability • Repeat prescriptions • **Communication**
Protocols/guidelines *Bolam v Friern Barnet Hospital 1957**	• Standard setting • Clinical governance • The Bolam test • **Communication**
Outside product licensing	• Legal 'grey area' (e.g. subcutaneous methotrexate) • Clinical trials and special cases • Depends on circumstances • **Communication**

*Italics highlight legal cases that have tested specific aspects of care.   Corcoran (1999)

- The law does not recognize the concept of 'team liability' (Dimond, 2002).
- All documents are potentially legal documents, including a patient-monitoring card.
- The NHS now has a responsibility to 'learn from experience'. Specific targets have been set to reduce levels of litigation (DoH, 2000a; National Patient Safety Agency, 2002).

There are areas of vulnerability and these are set out in Table 6.2. As can be seen from this table 'communication' is the identified factor that has been attributed to many failures in care.

What monitoring regimen should be used?

There is evidence that monitoring guidelines and practice vary from department to department and even within departments (Kay and Pullar, 1993). This variation not only relates to the frequency of monitoring, but also to which tests are done and the action to be taken in the event of abnormal results. Rheumatologists' practice has developed through a number of routes (Comer et al., 1995):

- general or consensus views (60%)
- clinical training (48%)
- pharmaceutical companies (48%)
- scientific literature (small minority – percentage not listed).

The British Society of Rheumatology (BSR, 2000) and the American College of Rheumatology have both produced drug-monitoring guidelines (ACR, 1996) that are designed to be adapted for local use. Although nurses carry out a large proportion of monitoring, they have not been involved in the development of these national guidelines (Byrne, 1998).

There are a number of patient needs and service provision factors that should inform the decision on selecting the best monitoring regimen for patients and they have been highlighted earlier in this chapter.

Are all these tests absolutely necessary?

There is an ongoing debate in the literature, with claims that monitoring tests are performed too often in relation to the number of ADRs that occur, creating a financial and time burden for both patients and the NHS (Comer et al., 1995; Aletaha and Smolen, 2002). Comer et al. (1995)

found that between 34 and 50% of rheumatologists believed that it was feasible to increase the intervals between monitoring to more than one month. From their audit, they recommended that three-monthly monitoring after an initial stabilizing period would have identified seven out of eight of the late ADRs that occurred in their audit population.

Aletaha and Smolen (2002) question whether extended monitoring is costly without adding any benefit. They found that DMARD-related laboratory abnormalities occurred in 9% of treatment courses. All of these occurred within the first 4 months of treatment. They conclude that monitoring blood tests performed at weeks 2 and 4, then monthly for the first four months, and three- to six-monthly thereafter would detect up to 98.3% of laboratory abnormalities in a 'timely manner'. Monitoring should be more frequent after dosage increases. The exception to this is ciclosporin, which the authors recommended should have more frequent follow-up throughout the treatment course. It is worth noting that neither of these studies includes leflunomide or biologic therapies.

However, in a study involving 2170 patients receiving 3923 DMARD treatment courses, while agreeing that most adverse drug reactions occur during the first six months of therapy, the authors identified two late reactions with methotrexate (Grove et al., 2001). These were a case of thrombocytopenia at 9.4 months and one of leucopenia at 16.9 months in patients on a steady dose of the drug. They therefore recommended that monitoring of methotrexate should continue in the long term, but did not make any firm recommendations on frequency.

Do drug monitoring clinics need to be audited?

Yes, although the aims of the audit, frequency and specific aspects to be audited will vary according to local need. There is increasing pressure to demonstrate the value of care provided, and especially in clinical areas such as drug monitoring, which could be considered an area of clinical risk. Audit is invaluable in identifying strengths and weakness of an intervention and, as the previous paragraph highlights, there remain areas of discussion as to whether current monitoring regimens are effective or too rigorous.

Audit results will highlight changes that have affected the percentage of patients monitored according to the guidelines. An example of this includes an audit and re-audit undertaken by one of the authors using a shared-care monitoring regimen (Oliver, 1997, 1999, unpublished). Having set up monitoring guidelines, an initial audit was undertaken, which demonstrated only a moderate level of adherence to monitoring guidelines (74%). Practice nurses were seeing the patient, taking blood and recording the blood results in the monitoring booklet. A change in primary care (driven by an increase in monitoring requests from secondary care) resulted in most patients having to see the phlebotomist for their blood monitoring and recording of results. Training and telephone support were provided for the phlebotomists. The re-audit demonstrated an improvement in adherence to guidelines (97.5%) despite the loss of the practice nurse time. However, there had been a 'safety net loss' because in nine cases patients were not having their blood results compared with previous results to identify a 'trend' in results.

The results of the audit will depend on what aspects of management are audited. It may be necessary to assess the level of work, skill mix and expertise of practitioners undertaking monitoring clinics, or the amount of time spent on drug monitoring as opposed to disease activity assessments, highlighting the need for additional nursing resource.

Conclusions

There are a number of issues that need to be considered when managing drug-monitoring clinics. The number of patients on long-term medications has risen expotentially. As a result, a variety of models of drug monitoring have been used, many using specialist nursing expertise. Supplementary prescribing will allow appropriately trained nurses and pharmacists using clinical management plans to prescribe treatments and alter drug dosages (DoH, 2003a).

Due to the increased awareness of clinical risk and clinical governance issues, the provision of monitoring clinics has become an area of interest in all healthcare initiatives. Healthcare providers will be interested in developing strategies that improve concordance with treatments and monitoring regimens. Rheumatology monitoring clinics have been at the forefront of patient empowerment and improving concordance with therapies. An important aspect has been the extensive educational support that patients receive before starting treatment and the use of a patient-held (or shared-care) monitoring record. Healthcare policies support the need to ensure that patients are empowered to manage their disease, are provided with the opportunity to give true 'informed consent' and have sufficient access to appropriate support and advice (DoH, 2001e). Many of the aspects discussed are already an integral part of rheumatology drug-monitoring clinics.

In conclusion, the provision of drug-monitoring clinics must be carefully planned, paying particular attention to the needs of the patients, supporting infrastructures (especially within primary care), guidelines used, provision of facilities and nursing expertise.

Chapter 7

The immune system and new treatments

Susan Oliver

Introduction

Much of the nursing assessment and care administered to a patient requires the practitioner to have knowledge of the immune processes and the subsequent problems faced if the immune response is altered or compromised. Healthcare professionals are aware of the principles of immunity in practical terms, but there is rarely a need for close scrutiny of the underlying theoretical concepts. The actual principles of an 'immune response' are assumed and the foundations of that knowledge rarely require testing when caring for patients. However, in the past decade, research has revealed fascinating insights into diseases of the immune system. With this research have come new treatments with the potential to block or 'disarm' cell interactions in the early stages of an immune response. These potentially powerful interventions have raised awareness of many autoimmune diseases and raised expectation that in the next decade there will be more effective treatments for autoimmune diseases. For the purpose of this discussion we are focusing on the mechanisms involved in autoimmune disease and new therapeutic agents developed specifically to target the early process of an immune response.

Using rheumatoid arthritis (RA) as an example, this chapter gives a simple explanation of an autoimmune disease and highlights some of the new therapies, how they work and the evidence supporting their use and potential benefits.

One of the earliest specific cytokines (powerful chemical messengers) that has undergone extensive research in this area is tumour necrosis factor alpha (TNFα), one of many cytokines involved in a normal inflammatory response. Following research identifying the role of cytokines it became possible to develop therapies to attempt to block them from playing their part in activating a cell response. The role of new cytokine-blocking agents such as anti-TNFα and a more recent treatment option, interleukin-1 receptor antagonist (IL-1ra), are addressed in the treatment of RA. There are three anti-TNFα blocking agents licensed for treating RA (adalimumab, etanercept and infliximab). There are a number of other diseases that may benefit from biologic therapies (see Table 7.2 on page 135).

This chapter discusses the theoretical aspects of targeted therapies and research evidence. The practical aspects of caring for patients receiving treatment are discussed in Chapter 8. This chapter includes:

- An overview of autoimmune disease and the role of cytokines and immunoglobulins.
- The action of new targeted therapies in the treatment of inflammatory joint disease with a specific emphasis on RA.
- Research evidence.

The immune response

The function of the immune system is to protect the body from attack or damage caused by micro-organisms. These micro-organisms could be bacteria, viruses, fungi or parasites. In the past, we were taught that there were two types of immune mechanisms: the innate or natural immunity, and the acquired or adaptive immunity (Table 7.1). Natural immunity is a non-specific rapid response and is not dependent on the body identifying the specific foreign organisms. Adaptive immunity is highly specific, relying on the body's ability to recognize the 'invader' and launch a targeted response based on clear recognition of the make-up of the organism.

Natural (innate) immunity prevents entry of micro-organisms into tissues using mechanical barriers, skin surfaces, mucous membranes and antibacterial substances in secretions. They do not become more efficient on repeated exposure but respond in the same way to all micro-organisms. Other aspects of this response occur by phagocytosis (the ingestion and killing of micro-organisms by specialist cells called phagocytes). This type of immune response is usually localized, for example inflammation around a break in the skin in response to micro-organisms crossing the normal immune barrier.

Acquired (adaptive) immunity is based on the memory of the immune system and its ability to recognize previous invaders. When the body recognizes a micro-organism that has previously 'invaded' the body the normal result is a 'specific and targeted response' to the invader. This system relies on the body recognizing 'self' and 'non-self' or invader cells.

Although these two types of immune response appear clear-cut and distinct, there are significant aspects of an immune response that are interrelated. This chapter focuses on the ability of the immune system to recognize an antigen or 'non-self' organism and launch a specific response.

Table 7.1 Acquired and active immunity

Acquired (adaptive) immunity	Active (innate) immunity
• Requires immune system 'memory' • Response slower than active immunity but specific target attack based upon previous exposure to antigen	• Normal protective immune mechanisms • Response does not alter despite repeated 'attacks'
• Immunity based on previous exposure	• Specific human immunity – present at birth (natural immunity to other species diseases, e.g. cowpox) • Genetic predisposition to some diseases, e.g cystic fibrosis
• Immunological recognition (antigen recognition)	• Skin, mucous membranes
• Discriminates between self and non-self	• Antibacterial secretions – tears, saliva
• Specific target response – recognize as foreign micro-organism/antigen	• Ciliary activity – upward flow of secretions – bronchial tree
• Reacts to 'invaders' by the production of specific antibodies (immunoglobulins)	• Coughing, vomiting
• Cellular basis of immune response – lymphocytes, T cells and B cells • Phagocytes also act on cell-mediated responses ingesting antigen and breaking down	• Skin – broken skin results in increased blood supply, increased capillary permeability allowing pooling of tissues, and non-specific ingestion of antigens (phagocytosis)
• Macrophages or lymphocytes present antigen to T cells and B cells	

The immune system

The immune system is a vast and fascinating topic. There is now a much greater understanding of the complex cell interactions that occur to produce an efficient immune system. In the past decade, research has revealed the pathways of human immune responses and the specific cell interactions. This has resulted in new treatments that are more specifically 'designed' to target key aspects of the immune process.

A number of chronic illnesses are known to have an autoimmune component, resulting in self-destruction of vital tissues. The consequences of the disease will depend on what tissues are damaged as a result of the body's 'malfunction'. Rheumatoid arthritis is a good example of an autoimmune disease. In RA, an abnormal immune response is 'triggered' by the immune system's faulty recognition of the 'self' molecules (such as immunoglobulin G). The body recognizes 'self' as 'foreign' and, in the example of RA, this results in a targeted response on the synovial tissue that lines all moveable joints. Similar responses are seen in other 'faulty' immune responses, for example the immune system of a patient with diabetes mellitus recognizes pancreatic cells as 'foreign' and as a result triggers an immune response that causes cell damage to the pancreas.

To understand immunity it is useful to think of the immune system as working as an army (Isenberg and Morrow, 1995). An antigen is a foreign substance that invades the body and the body's response to antigens or 'foreign' invaders is to launch a response from lymphocytes. Lymphocytes are a type of white blood cell that originates in bone marrow and initially are called 'stem cells'. These stem cells are similar to new young recruits, and the bone marrow can be thought of as a major headquarters and recruitment centre. The young stem cells are developed and trained as general soldiers. These general soldiers are called 'B'-lymphocyte cells. Some of these general soldiers are sent to base camps around the body.

The base camps are situated in lymphoid tissue in the tonsils, adenoids, lymph nodes, spleen, lymphatic vessels and patches of lymphoid tissue in the intestines (Figure 7.1).

T and B cells

T and B cells are mature lymphocytes and are essential in the normal immune system, recognizing and responding to 'invasions' by foreign invaders such as antigens. The system is very efficient, with cells being able to travel from lymphoid tissue in the 'base camps' to other areas. Communication between various lymphoid camps is achieved via the

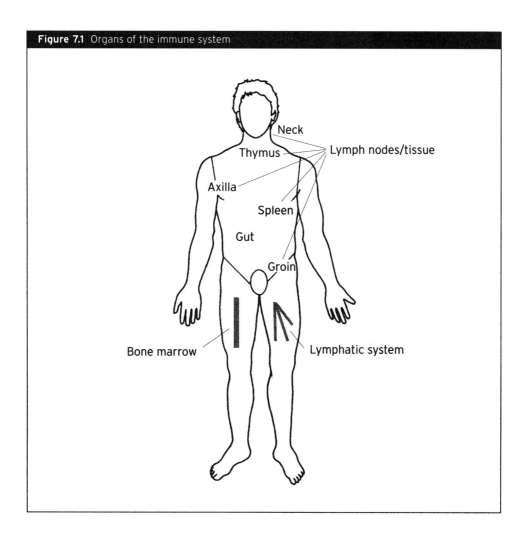

Figure 7.1 Organs of the immune system

lymphatic system. (One quarter of all developed T-lymphocyte cells are present in the lymphoid tissues.)

Some of these stem cells are sent to train as specialist cells in the thymus gland. The thymus is also lymphoid tissue and can be thought of as an 'elite' training camp. Stem cells from here are then called 'T'-lymphocyte cells.

There are now two specific types of lymphocyte cells to remember: T cells and B cells. Although T cells and B cells have their own unique roles in arming the immune system, they also have some common characteristics (Figure 7.2). Both T and B cells are capable of 'clonal expansion', that

Figure 7.2 Common characteristics of B cells and T cells

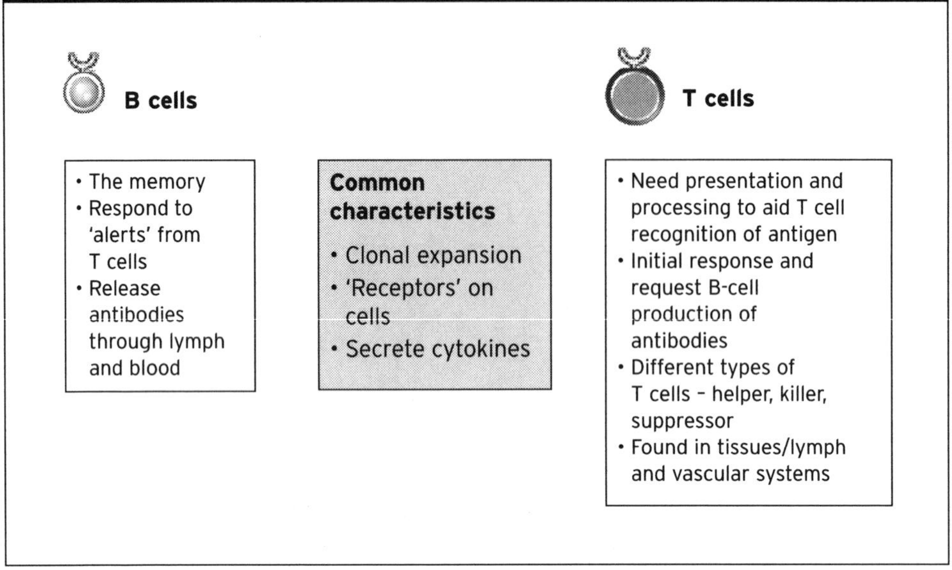

B cells

- The memory
- Respond to 'alerts' from T cells
- Release antibodies through lymph and blood

Common characteristics

- Clonal expansion
- 'Receptors' on cells
- Secrete cytokines

T cells

- Need presentation and processing to aid T cell recognition of antigen
- Initial response and request B-cell production of antibodies
- Different types of T cells – helper, killer, suppressor
- Found in tissues/lymph and vascular systems

is the ability to reproduce themselves rapidly when needed. They have 'receptors' that enable good communication and contact with antigens (foreign invaders). Another important role of T and B cells is the ability to secrete potent chemical messengers (cytokines) that trigger a response from other cells, particularly in response to a 'foreign invader' or antigen. Cytokines can be secreted by T or B cells, although it is predominantly the role of the T cells. A clear difference between the two cells is that T cells need antigens to be 'presented' to them in a specific way (see below).

Antigen-presenting cells

T cells will identify an antigen when an antigen-presenting cell (APC) comes into contact with the T cell and presents an antigen to it. This antigen is carried within a specific binding groove of a major histocompatibility complex (MHC) molecule that is transported to the surface of the APC. The type of antigen (e.g. virus, bacterium) will determine whether it is presented to the T cell by a type I or type II MHC molecule.

This chapter does not give a detailed explanation of MHC molecules and how they work, but what is important to understand is that antigen presentation by the MHC system is an essential process in alerting the lymphocyte cells to launch an appropriate attack. (For further information on MHCs, see Hoffbrand and Pettit, 1993.) Examples of APCs include B cells and macrophages. One of the most significant roles of macrophages is to work as APCs, although they play numerous roles as part of the immune army. They are distributed throughout the body in tissues and blood, and have the potential to consume passing antigens and immune complexes by phagocytosis. Other cells in the immune system can also undertake this role. When the macrophage works as an APC it uses enzymes partially to break down the proteins in the antigen to smaller peptides before presenting these to the T cells.

The way in which the APC presents the antigen to the T cell will also influence the type of response that the T cell should make to the antigen. This is a complex process, but the chief point to remember is that a T cell can launch a different response depending on the antigen presented.

In humans, the MHC is also referred to as human leucocyte antigen (HLA). The HLA system determines which antigens are recognized by an individual, and it varies from person to person. Rheumatoid arthritis is strongly linked to the HLA-DRB1 region of the MHC class II complex. This complex association continues to be an area of interest in research to identify the cause and processes involved in autoimmune disease. Molecules of the MHC class II complex present the antigen to T-helper cells. The activation of T-helper cells with a specific marker attached (called CD4) induces a cytokine response as well as an antibody response from the B cells (Choy and Panayi, 2001). Although there are other immune cells involved in this response, it is important for this discussion to focus on the T-helper cell.

Cytokines

The response that the T cell launches is the release of a powerful chemical messenger or cytokine. Monocytes, macrophages, fibroblasts and T cells can release numerous cytokines on stimulation.

Cytokines are proteins or glycoproteins that deliver important intercellular messages regulating chronic inflammation and tissue damage in RA. Each cytokine has a specific role within the immune system. Such roles can include activating (inducing) an acute phase response, increasing cell adhesion, cell growth and production of destructive enzymes in RA. In recent years, research has identified an increasing number of cytokines, with approximately 150 now documented (Dinarello and Moldawer, 2000). Some of these cytokines are grouped into families, such as interleukin-1 (IL-1), TNFα, interleukin-6 (IL-6) and granulocyte–macrophage colony-stimulating factor (GM-CSF). These cytokines are specifically mentioned because they are present in abundance in inflamed joints.

The cytokine or messenger can be released in the blood or lymphatic system, and once it is released it needs to 'lock into' a T-cell receptor (TCR) (Figure 7.3). It can then launch a number of different responses. Sometimes the T cell will recognize the need to launch a response from a

---

Figure 7.3 T-cell receptors and interactions

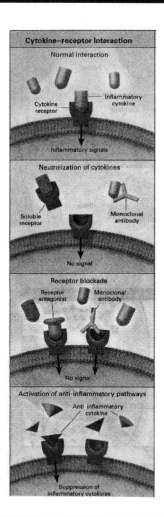

Normal inflammatory response with cytokine locking into T-cell receptor, activating an inflammatory response

Neutralization or 'disarming' of cytokines by preventing activation. Monoclonal antibody prevents activation

Receptor agonist displacing cytokine and thus preventing activation of inflammatory response

There are pro- and anti-inflammatory cytokines. The balance between these cytokines can be disrupted as in the case of RA, where pro-inflammatory cytokines result in an increase in the normal inflammatory response

---

Reproduced from Choy EHS, Panayi GS (2001) Cytokine pathways and joint inflammation in rheumatoid arthritis. New England Journal of Medicine 344: 907–915.

'suppressor' T cell that causes a reduction of the normal attack or immune response, resulting in anti-inflammatory cytokine responses. It is this process that tells the T cell army to 'stand down' when an antigen is no longer functioning or has been adequately 'disarmed', signalling that the immune response has been effective and should stop.

Immunoglobulins (antibodies)

B-lymphocyte cells, although less highly specialized than T-lymphocyte cells, are the memory of the immune system. B cells can be thought of as the intelligence corp of an army and, as mentioned earlier, are based mainly in the lymphoid tissues around the body. They have the ability to remember many previous antigens (foreign invaders) and have a tailor-made immune response that can destroy the antigen. The B cells will respond quickly to requests from T cells when they recognize the initial attack from an antigen. The B-cell memory results in a tailor-made decisive 'bullet' or attack on the antigen released through the lymphatic or blood system. This tailor-made (bullet) response is an immunoglobulin (antibody).

An immunoglobulin is almost always a Y-shaped structure. Understanding the significance of this shape to the way an immunoglobulin functions can help us to understand how some of the new treatments work to control autoimmune diseases. Part of the structure is 'constant' and part is 'flexible' (i.e. changeable). The V or top part of the Y shape is the flexible section and is where the antigen binds when it is trapped by the immunoglobulin. It is this section that can be manipulated in the laboratory when developing new drugs. To understand this further we need to focus on the normal mechanism of action of the immunoglobulin.

When a B cell recognizes an antigen it sends out an immunoglobulin made specifically to match that antigen. There is a precise area on the V section of the immunoglobulin that has tiny 'jigsaw-like' shapes cut out of it, and these cut-out areas match exactly the shape of the antigen. This acts like a lock and key, or two jigsaw pieces fitting together (Figure 7.4). The region of the antigen that the immunoglobulin recognizes is called an epitope. Many different potential antibody-producing B cells pre-exist in the body, each with the ability to make an antibody of a different specificity. If an immunoglobulin and antigen are perfectly matched, they are said to have a shared 'epitope'. This is an effective immune response. On binding antigen, the B cell is activated to divide and produce identical cells which produce identical antibodies to the specific antigen. If a B cell encounters an antigen it has not seen before, it will need to produce a new immunoglobulin (antibody) specifically to match that antigen, and then

divide and produce more identical cells producing identical immunoglobulin. The B cell will then memorize the antigen characteristics so that a
more specific targeted response can be used next time the antigen invades
the body.

Figure 7.4 Antigens and immunoglobulins

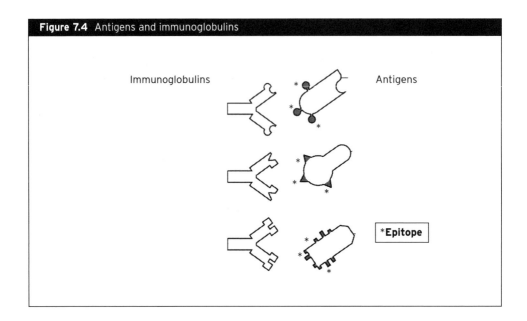

Both T cells and B cells are essential in the normal immune response.
Recalling that the T-helper cell needs to have a specific antigen presented
to it by an APC and MHC, it is now possible to clarify the chain of events
in RA.

One theory is that, at some point, an antigen response is made against
a foreign or self-protein which triggers an inflammatory cascade. The particular antigen involved has not been identified. It could be a foreign
antigen such as a bacterium or virus, or a self-antigen such as collagen or
IgG. Antigen is broken into small peptide fragments within APCs before
becoming bound to MHC class II molecules. Only certain peptides will
bind to the MHC class II molecules, depending on the particular form of
the MHC class II molecule and the size and amino acid sequence of the
peptide fragments. MHC class II genes exist as many different variants.
Certain individuals with particular MHC class II variants are more susceptible to RA. All MHC class II modules associated with RA have a
common region where they bind to antigenic peptides. This has led to the

suggestion that these particular MHC variants bind and present a peptide that is able to trigger RA.

T-cell receptors can be circulating in soluble form (that is, circulating in the blood and lymphatic system) or tissue-bound (as in the synovial tissues). When a T-cell 'locks into' a TCR, this activates the release of other cytokines that enhance the inflammatory response. The release of these pro-inflammatory cytokines (interleukin 1, interleukin 6, interleukin 8 and GM-CSF) is often termed the 'inflammatory cascade' (see Figure 7.5). This is because they enhance the action of the inflammatory response in the synovial tissues, causing an increase in synovial cell proliferation, increased cell infiltration and permeability, as well as changes in bony modelling (Maini, 2002).

Figure 7.5 Inflammatory cascade

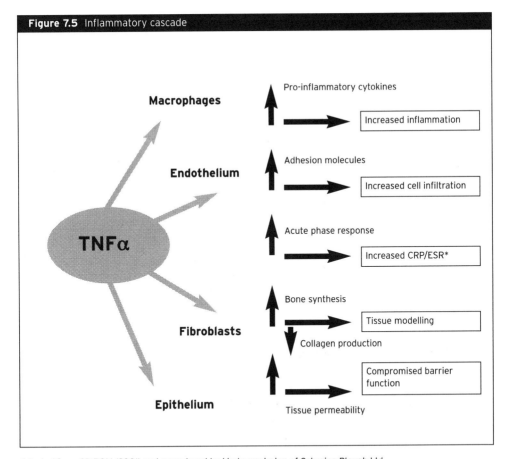

Adapted from CD ROM (2001) and reproduced by kind permission of Schering Plough Ltd.
*CRP: C-reactive protein   ESR: erythrocyte sedimentation rate

The development of cytokine-blocking therapies is the result of biological technology that 'designs' the 'blocking' mechanism. This mimicking of the immune process enables the disarming of the normal 'lock-and-key' response and thus the 'inflammatory cascade' fails to be activated. These new targeted therapies are sometimes referred to as 'biologics', as they are biologically engineered (Oliver and Mooney, 2002).

Targeted therapies – an overview

The recognition of TNFα and its role in the inflammatory cascade led researchers to focus on the development of an antibody to 'lock into' or 'block' the cytokine from connecting to its cell-surface receptor. The result of this research is a number of new therapies, focused on the two specific cytokines implicated in instigating the inflammatory cascade in RA, TNFα and IL-1.

Pro-inflammatory cytokines

The characteristic signs seen in RA (tender, swollen and painful joints with active synovitis) are the result of pro-inflammatory cytokines inducing an inflammatory cascade (Figure 7.5), and the two dominant cytokines involved are TNFα and IL-1. These cytokines need to lock onto specific receptors on the surface of cells, such as those in synovial tissue. Early cytokine identification documented specific cytokines as responsible for either pro- or anti-inflammatory responses. As knowledge of cytokines has developed, it has been suggested that specific cytokines recognized as having a pro-inflammatory action may have other, perhaps more sophisticated or inter-related, responses, depending on other cytokine interactions or disease processes.

Therapeutic options

The success of these biologic therapies in treating RA has led to research into the benefits of cytokine-blocking agents in other forms of inflammatory joint disease. Early research with infliximab has shown promising results in the treatment of spondyloarthropathies such as psoriatic arthritis and ankylosing spondylitis (Ritchlin, 2001; Braun et al., 2002; Kirkham, 2003). Interestingly, research studies to date into Crohn's disease have demonstrated significant benefit from treatment with infliximab, but standard doses of etanercept failed to achieve the same levels of benefit (Hommes, 2003). This may be as a result of bolus dosing regimens or dosage ranges, or it may be related to differences in the two therapies. However, etanercept has demonstrated significant benefit in the treatment of juvenile idiopathic arthritis (JIA) (Lovell et al., 2003).

Research has now extended to other chronic diseases (Table 7.2), and it is likely that other medical specialities will wish to benefit from the research evidence and clinical experience that practitioners in the field of rheumatology have gained in the use of biologic therapies.

Table 7.2 Current or potential treatments with biologic therapies

Specialist area	Disease areas using or researching biologic therapies
Gastroenterology	Inflammatory bowel disease Crohn's disease
Ophthalmology	Uveitis Scleritis Behçet's disease
Dermatology	Psoriasis Psoriatic arthritis Eczema Melanoma
Hepatology	Hepatitis C
Nephrology	Glomerulonephritis Vasculitic disease causing renal damage (e.g. Wegner's)
Respiratory	Asthma Rhinitis Chronic obstructive pulmonary disease (COPD)

Anti-TNFα therapies

There are three different anti-TNFα treatments (infliximab, adalimumab and etanercept), and two types of T-cell receptor for TNFα to lock into: p55 and p75. These are specific receptors for TNFα cytokines. The difference between these two distinct receptors is their molecular size (Dinarello, 2003). Infliximab and adalimumab block both p55 and p75 receptors, whereas etanercept blocks p55 receptors only. Infliximab is an engineered antibody against TNFα and can block soluble and tissue-bound receptors. Adalimumab has similar properties to infliximab. Etanercept is an engineered soluble receptor molecule that interferes with the binding of TNFα and blocks cell-surface receptors. It also has the potential to bind to a cytokine called lymphotoxin alpha as well as to TNFα. The clinical relevance of etanercept blocking the cytokine lympotoxin alpha is not yet known, although it is thought that this may be relevant in the treatment of juvenile rheumatoid arthritis, as lymphotoxin alpha is present in inflamed synovial tissue in this disease (Pisetsky, 2000).

It is important at this point to clarify the role of TNFα in one additional respect. As the name implies TNFα has a role in causing death or necrosis of malignant or pre-malignant cells within the body. Blocking this process has the theoretical possibility of allowing malignant or pre-malignant cells to develop. However, in all post-marketing surveillance and evidence to date, this theoretical risk has not been proven. Interpreting the risk of anti-TNFα treatments and malignancy in RA are complex. This is partly due to the additional risk of malignancy attributed to aggressive disease, disease duration and the use of toxic treatments (e.g. cyclophosphamide, ciclosporin, azathioprine, methotrexate).

Etanercept and infliximab

The development of anti-TNFα therapies has given patients an opportunity of disease suppression and improved quality of life. At the time of going to press there are three licensed anti-TNFα therapies that have been developed to treat active RA. These therapies are etanercept, infliximab and adalimumab.

Etanercept and infliximab have been reviewed by the National Institute for Clinical Excellence published guidance for the use of these therapies in RA (NICE, 2002a). In addition, etanercept has been reviewed for the treatment of children and young adults with JIA (NICE, 2002a). The relevance of NICE reviews and publication of guidance are discussed in Chapters 2, 8 and 12.

Adalimumab

A third anti-TNFα treatment (adalimumab) has not yet been reviewed by NICE. Adalimumab is a fully human anti-TNFα treatment that blocks the TCRs p55 and p75 in soluble and tissue-bound forms. Early published research data looks promising, with significant improvement in disease activity for RA patients (Rau, 2003).

Interleukin-1 receptor antagonist therapy

IL-1 is a cytokine implicated in the inflammatory cascade and the subsequent mechanisms that lead to progressive joint destruction in RA. Anakinra is a recombinant form of the human IL-1Ra, an anti-inflammatory cytokine. Anakinra actively competes with IL-1, locking into the receptor and thus disarming the potential of the pro-inflammatory cytokine IL-1, which causes progressive joint destruction in RA. IL-1Ra is normally present in the body, but it is thought that patients with inflammatory joint disease have relatively low amounts of naturally occurring IL-1Ra, while the amount of IL-1 is high. This means that more IL-1 cytokine molecules are able to lock into the receptors resulting in an inflammatory response (Jiang et al., 2000). The early evidence suggests that anakinra reduces the rate of joint erosions and the signs and symptoms of RA (Bresnihan, 2001; Nuki, 2002). Anakinra provides an important therapeutic option for patients who have failed anti-TNFα therapies. Anakinra has been reviewed by NICE, and the NICE Technology Assessment Report should be published in 2003 (NICE, 2003b). For further analysis of the characteristics of biologics, see Table 7.3.

Biologics/targeted therapies – research evidence

Etanercept and infliximab treatments have demonstrated a significant impact on improving the lives of patients with RA as well as reducing the rate of joint erosions (Furst et al., 2002). Keane et al. (2001) state that 147 000 patients have received anti-TNFα treatments worldwide, and the data suggest that 70% of patients have a good response to anti-TNFα therapy (Emery et al., 1999). It is an expensive treatment compared to conventional treatment; however, for the patient with RA, the most important factor, potentially affecting the long-term impact of the disease, has been the reduction in erosions to joints on radiographic evidence (Maini et al., 1999).

In the process of educating, assessing and managing patients with new therapies, it is essential that practitioners have a clear understanding of the guidelines, specific issues relating to each treatment and the mechanisms of action. In this section we focus on the research evidence relevant to the clinical issues in caring for patients receiving targeted therapies.

The initial research work on new treatments usually focuses on the safety and efficacy aspects of a new drug. This brief overview of research evidence is based on the early data as well as recent research evidence. It is essential to remember that selection, treatment groups, dosages and

Table 7.3 Targeted therapies and characteristics

Drug	Properties	Administration	Length of action
Anakinra (Kineret) Licensed for RA to be administered concomitantly with methotrexate	Interleukin-1 receptor antagonist Human antibody – DNA technology using *Escherichia coli* Actively competes with IL-1Ra by blocking IL-1 receptors	100 mg by daily subcutaneous injection	Maximum plasma concentration 3–7 hours after injection Half-life 4–6 hours
Adalimumab (Humira) Licensed for RA Can be administered as mono or combination therapy with methotrexate	Anti-TNFα Human antibody biologically engineered using *Escherichia coli* Blocks T-cell receptors in soluble and tissue-bound forms	40 mg subcutaneous injection given every two weeks. Can also be prescribed weekly when response is suboptimal in monotherapy	Half-life 10–18 days
Etanercept (Enbrel) Licensed for: RA, psoriatic arthritis and juvenile idiopathic arthritis	Anti-TNFα Human antibody grafted to human antibody. Binds TNFa and blocks the interaction with cell-surface receptors. Etanercept also blocks lymphotoxin alpha	Adult dose: 25 mg twice weekly by subcutaneous injection Paediatric dose: 4 mg/kg of body weight to a maximum of 25 mg twice-weekly per injection	Maximum concentration approximately 48 hours after a single dose Half-life 70 hours
Infliximab (Remicade) Licensed for RA, Crohn's disease, ankylosing spondylitis. To be administered concomitantly with methotrexate	Anti-TNFα Mouse and human antibody. Blocks T-cell receptors soluble and tissue-bound. Does not block lymphotoxins	Infliximab administered at a dose of 3 mg/kg of body weight for RA Infusion regimen of 0 (first infusion), then 2 weeks after first infusion and then 6 weeks after first infusion, then 8-weekly thereafter. One initial dose of 5 mg/kg for active and fistulizing Crohn's disease. If good response, two choices of treatment: maintenance or readministration when disease flares Active Crohn's: maintenance treatment at 0 (first infusion), then 2 and 6 weeks after first infusion, followed by 8-weekly; readministration: one treatment when disease recurs Fistulizing Crohn's: 2 and 6 weeks after first infusion; repeat at 2 and 6 weeks after first infusion Ankylosing spondylitis (dose 5 mg/kg) 2 and 6 weeks after the first infusion, then every 6–8 weeks. If no response at 6 weeks no additional treatment advised Unlicensed indication for psoratic arthritis and at dose regimens varying from 3 mg/kg to 5 mg/kg of body weight	Terminal half-life range between 8.0 and 9.5 days

Source: Summary of Product Characteristics:
Amgen (April 2002), Schering Plough (May 2003), Wyeth (May 2003), Abbott Laboratories (October 2003).

duration of disease, number of previous treatments allowed, age and sex of treatment groups, etc., are all details that will vary in each clinical trial. These differences (or variables) have the potential to affect the overall final research findings and need to be thoroughly evaluated when reviewing a research paper. However, the aim of this section is to focus on providing an overview and not a meta-analysis or systematic review of the research evidence related to patients receiving biologic therapies.

It is important to remember that this is an area that is rapidly evolving, and reviewing evidence is an ongoing process, with regular publications highlighting the latest research. Practitioners need to update their knowledge of latest research evidence on a regular basis. This is of added importance in evolving areas of practice where patients have regular access to the Internet, and much of the latest information is readily available to them in easily understood formats.

Measures used to assess benefit of treatment in RA - disease activity

There is a need to have an effective method of assessing the patient's response to treatment. This response should be measurable, relevant to the patient group and reliable. For an in-depth discussion on outcome measures, refer to Chapter 5.

When evaluating a potential improvement or deterioration in the disease (or any research intervention), it is important to have a clear understanding of what outcomes are to be measured and whether they have any value in demonstrating a change. A greater consistency in the interpretation of research results can be achieved if there is a clear agreement about what counts as an objective improvement to the disease process. In the field of rheumatology, a consensus on what constitutes an improvement in signs and symptoms of RA has been achieved. However, there is a difference between the comprehensive range of information collated as part of a full research project and outcome measures used to assess benefit in routine clinical practice. For this reason we discuss the research data collected followed by a detailed review of data collected in the clinical care setting.

A significant proportion of research work is undertaken in the USA and therefore it is essential to understand the research outcome criteria as defined by the American College of Rheumatology (ACR). The ACR (Arnett et al., 1988) set out criteria that are routinely used to measure levels of response to treatment (Table 7.4).

For the ACR criteria, level of response is determined based on the reduction in number of tender joints and the number of swollen joints and

Table 7.4 ACR criteria for measuring level of response to treatments

1   Number of tender joints (of 28 assessed using EULAR core data-set)*
2   Number of swollen joints (of 28 assessed using EULAR core data-set)*
3   Health Assessment Questionnaire (HAQ)
4   Patient assessment of disease activity/global health
    (using a visual analogue scale, VAS)*
5   Patient assessment of pain (using a VAS)*
6   Physician global assessment (using a VAS)*
7   Erythrocyte sedimentation rate (ESR) or C-reactive protein (CRP) blood tests

These measures are used in routine joint assessments in many clinic settings and are well validated (van Riel and Scott, 2000).

at least three of the remaining five variables. If a 20% improvement on baseline measurements is obtained in tender and swollen joints and at least three of the five ACR core set measures, the patient is said to have achieved an ACR 20 improvement (Felson et al., 1995). The ACR response criteria for the ACR 50 and ACR 70 applies in the same way, that is, if the patient has achieved a 50% improvement on baseline assessment in the measurements outlined above, they will be said to have achieved an ACR 50% improvement in their disease activity.

In Europe, much of the European League Against Rheumatism (EULAR) core data-set is used to assess the benefit of biologic therapies in the clinical care setting. The EULAR core data-set includes 28 tender and swollen joint count assessments, including two visual analogue scales (VASs), one for pain and one for general global assessment of disease activity. The data-set also forms part of the ACR criteria for identifying response to treatment (Table 7.4). Most of these measures are used to form a composite score called the disease activity score (DAS). The DAS is the assessment criterion that the British Society for Rheumatology (BSR) Guidelines use as part of the selection process for prescribing anti-TNFα treatment (BSR Working Party, 2000).

The measures that form part of the essential data collection for adherence to NICE guidance (2002a) include the DAS. The score is based on:

- 28 tender joint count
- 28 swollen joint count
- patient's global assessment of disease activity (using a 100 mm VAS)
- blood taken to measure erythrocyte sedimentation rate (ESR).

There is a statistical calculation weighting different components of the measures. The DAS is calculated using a modified scoring system:

DAS = $0.555\sqrt{}$(28 tender joints) + $0.284\sqrt{}$(28 swollen joints) + 0.70 ln (ESR) + 0.0142 (patient global assessment).

Most nurses and physicians have access to computer software programs or hand-held DAS calculators to enable rapid calculation of the total DAS. The EULAR 28 joint count is recognized as valid and reliable in measuring changes in disease activity in a clinical setting (Scott et al., 1995). The DAS has been recognized as one of the regular assessments required to evaluate benefit of treatment when assessing patients receiving biologics.

The assessment of a DAS response to treatment includes two components. One is the eligibility for treatment and the second is the benefit achieved following at least three months of treatment. Patients who fulfil the inclusion criteria and have a DAS of greater than 5.1 (measured at two time intervals a month apart) are eligible for treatment. The criteria to remain on treatment are that there should be an improvement relative to the past DAS scores (benefit of > 1.2) or improvement to a level of disease activity (DAS < 3.2). The BSR criteria for improvement in disease activity can be seen in Table 7.5.

Table 7.5 BSR criteria for assessment of disease activity score (DAS) and benefit of treatment

DAS assessed at two time points one month apart before commencing treatment	Score should be > 5.1
Improvement in DAS	• Relative to past score DAS > 1.2 • Improvement to a low level of disease activity DAS < 3.2

The DAS has provided an objective tool to measure the benefits of treatment. However, as with all assessment tools, there are weaknesses that fail to identify specific patient groups. It is therefore possible that at times the prescribing physician will treat a patient with biologic therapies despite the fact that they fail the criteria for treatment. Some of the possible reasons could include:

• Patients with multiple joint replacements (no swollen/tender joints evident).
• Features of extra-articular disease (e.g. significant lung involvement from RA lung). Patients with extra-articular features have been shown to have a higher rate of mortality (Turesson et al., 1999).

• Evidence of significant erosive disease despite low DAS (e.g. multiple joint replacements and need for life-threatening surgery, e.g. cervical surgery; Casey and Crockard, 1995).

In the UK, the BSR set out inclusion and exclusion criteria for treatment with anti-TNFα treatments (BSR Working Party, 2000). The BSR guidelines are an integral part of the NICE guidance for treatment of patients with RA. Similar criteria have been set by the British Paediatric Rheumatology Group (BPRG, 2000) to be used when assessing children and young people with JIA. NICE guidance (2002a) has accepted the BPRG guidelines for the use of etanercept in JIA. Although there are limitations to the selection criteria for biologic therapies, these guidelines provided an effective starting point and, like all guidelines, as practice and experience develop the guidelines should be reviewed to take into account the problems identified.

Research continues into the most effective methods of administering treatment, with particular focus on the optimum dosing regimens and intervals between treatment. A study evaluating dose titration using the DAS 28 found marked variations in the required dose of anti-TNFα needed to sustain a therapeutic benefit (den Broeder et al., 2002). Patients in this study had received a full year of anti-TNFα treatment at entry. It was for this reason that the study aimed to maintain or reduce the individual patient's DAS at entry. This small study provides some insight into possible developments in biologic treatments. Detailed discussions on the assessment, administration and management of patients receiving biologic therapies is set out in Chapter 8.

Many patients currently eligible for treatment are those who have had significant joint destruction and the subsequent consequences of long-standing disease. Patients with RA have been shown to have similar risk and mortality to patients with cardiovascular disease and non-Hodgkin's lymphoma (Pincus and Callahan, 1993). In the next few years, given effective data collection and the demonstration of continued long-term benefits of biologic therapies, it may be that healthcare purchasers will recognize the potential overall benefits to patients, society and the healthcare system, and increase access to treatment as a result. As nurses, assessing patients, collecting data and providing care, we have a role and responsibility in the long-term provision of care.

Ankylosing spondylitis

Infliximab has recently been licensed for the treatment of patients with ankylosing spondylitis (AS) who have severe axial symptoms and demonstrate evidence of high inflammatory markers of disease activity (e.g. C-reactive protein, CRP). There are additional clinical measures that need to be used to assess disease activity in AS (Bath AS Disease Activity Index, BSDAI, and the Bath AS Functional Index, BASFI). For a detailed discussion on AS trials and future considerations on measures to assess therapeutic benefit of treatment, see van der Heijde et al. (2002). However, it is important to remember that, apart from these additional measures, many of the screening and assessment issues remain the same.

Benefits of treatment with biologics – disease activity

Current treatment with disease-modifying anti-rheumatic drugs

The treatment of RA relies heavily on the use of drugs such as non-steroidal anti-inflammatory drugs (NSAIDs), steroids, disease-modifying anti-rheumatic drugs (DMARDs), cytotoxic agents and, recently, the targeted therapies. Although this chapter uses RA as an example, other diseases known to have an autoimmune component have been shown to benefit from therapeutic interventions to reduce or block the normal immune responses (e.g. Crohn's disease). Many immunosuppressive therapies have evolved, sometimes without a clear understanding of the mechanisms that reduce the immune response. These treatments have focused on suppressing the immune system or modifying the disease process with DMARDs. The use of immunosuppressive agents, which have some effect on controlling the disease process, are not without a range of serious side effects and yet still fail to suppress the disease adequately (Tugwell et al., 2000). In AS, DMARDs and various immuno-suppressive agents have been found to be less effective than in the RA population (Sieper et al., 2002).

To recognize the full benefit of treatment with biologics, the results need to be compared with the benefits of treatment with traditional DMARDs. However, there are problems in comparing traditional DMARD therapy and the results of clinical trials using objective criteria such as the ACR or DAS assessments. Although in the past data have been collected on clinical measures, such as tender and swollen joint counts, it was not until recently that the DAS scoring system was used in research data. Much of the evidence available refers to ACR response criteria or individual factors measured and documented, for example an improvement in tender joint count score. The results are difficult to generalize from all the studies undertaken. Patients recruited varied from those with early RA to those with longstanding disease duration and patients on con-comitant therapies such as steroids. Time points for assessment, length of time assessed, varying dosage regimens (with or without a disease-modifying drug) and different methods and time frames for measuring radiological progression add to the complexities of making head to head comparisons. It is therefore not possible, and beyond the remit of this chapter, to provide a detailed analysis of comparisons between individual biologic therapies and traditional DMARD therapies.

The early research on anti-TNFα therapy began in 1992 with infliximab. The first drug (etanercept) was licensed for use in RA in 1998 and infliximab in 1999. These two drugs have now been widely used with approximately 121 000 patients (up to September 2001) prescribed etanercept and 271 000 patients treated with infliximab (up to February 2002) (Maini, 2002). The data for adalimumab is limited in this chapter, as to date only preliminary research data have been published.

Treatment with conventional DMARD therapies has been shown to reduce erosions and functional disability (Pincus et al., 2002). Yet it is clear that a significant proportion of patients fail to have their disease adequately controlled using standard treatments and there is a high rate of drug cessation due to toxicity or loss of efficacy (Pincus et al., 1992). Even so, in a 20-year follow-up study, where patients demonstrated effective disease control and reductions in erosions, 50% of patients required at least one (and some up to six) large joint replacements (Capell et al., 2001).

The potential risks of untreated RA have been shown to include joint destruction, work disability and premature mortality, as seen in 30–60% of patients (Pincus and Sokka 2001). In the past, complete remission has been an almost unachievable goal (Emery and Salmon, 1995). It remains to be seen whether this goal can now be achieved using biologic therapies. It will also be useful to build on early research which shows that prompt treatment for newly diagnosed patients with aggressive disease has the potential to prevent joint damage and subsequent deformity if used earlier in the course of the disease process.

The provision of effective treatments should consider:

- The long-term prognosis of patients who fail to have their disease actively controlled.
- The limit of therapeutic options for traditional disease-modifying drugs. Approximately 10% of DMARD treatments are continued for no longer than three years, with methotrexate having a slightly longer timespan than other drugs (Wolfe and Zwillich, 1998).
- The long-term side effects in patients who have failed all conventional therapies, remaining on steroids and anti-inflammatory drugs to reduce symptoms.
- The costs of disability to the patient, loss of work and increased risk of co-morbidity (Pincus and Callahan, 1993). Evidence highlights the link between increasing disability (as measured by the HAQ) and mortality

(Wolfe and Zwillich, 1998). HAQ scores are also predictive of work disability (Callahan et al., 1992).

- Potential reduction in emergency and routine hospital admissions.

Assessing measuring of disease activity – functional status

One essential element of measuring improvements relevant to the daily consequences for the patient is that of functional ability. The ACR classification for functional status in RA is set out in Table 7.6. This classification enables researchers to identify the level of functional ability of patients before and after treatment. A functional assessment tool frequently used is the HAQ. The HAQ is recognized as the 'gold standard' in the UK. The purpose of this section is to identify the changes measured pre- and post-treatment. However, for more detailed discussions on the HAQ and outcome measures see Chapter 5.

Functional ability as measured by the HAQ will vary in level of improvement achieved based on how much irreversible joint damage the individual patient has. Equally, in the author's experience, patients who have active disease already have a number of aids that remain in their home and they may continue to use them or continue to identify them as being used on the questionnaire despite experiencing a significant improvement in global health. The HAQ negatively scores the use of aids such as a walking stick, chair raisers, etc.

Table 7.6 American College of Rheumatology classification of functional status in RA*

Class	Criteria**
I	Able to perform usual activities of daily living (self-care, vocational, avocational)
II	Able to perform self-care and vocational activities, but limited in avocational activities
III	Able to perform self-care activities but limited in vocational and avocational activities
IV	Limited in ability to perform self-care, vocational and avocational activities

*In the UK, the Health Assessment Questionnaire would be used in a similar way to assess functional ability.
**Self-care includes: dressing, feeding, bathing, grooming and toileting; vocational activities include work, educational and/or homemaking activities; avocational activities include recreational and/or leisure activities.

The use of visual analogue scales to measure the patient's perceived pain and global health probably provides the greatest insight into the key factors that affect the individual's quality of life. The DAS core data-set captures elements of this information. Additional questionnaires such as the Short Form 36 (SF-36) are also collected as part of the data-set for the BSR Biologics Register (BSRBR) and this will be used to aid the assessment of overall improvement in health. Individuals with RA frequently report fatigue as a major symptom that has a dramatic effect on quality of life. One biologic research study for biologic therapies did include an outcome measure for fatigue (FACIT). Significant improvements (reduction in fatigue) were seen from baseline measurements in the treatment groups (Weinblatt et al., 2003).

Bandolier (2001) studied the rank order of the chronic diseases using the SF-36. The study identified musculoskeletal diseases as scoring a higher impact on quality of life than cardiovascular, neurology and gastrointestinal conditions.

Assessing disease activity - radiological changes

An additional measure that is becoming increasingly more important is the identification of radiological changes (such as joint erosions or joint

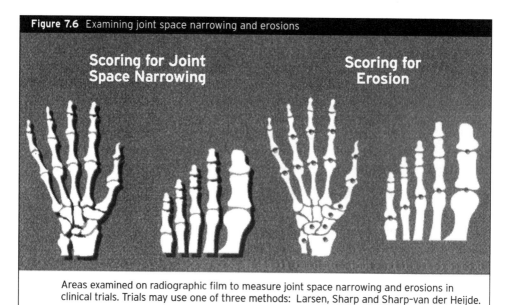

Figure 7.6 Examining joint space narrowing and erosions

Scoring for Joint Space Narrowing

Scoring for Erosion

Areas examined on radiographic film to measure joint space narrowing and erosions in clinical trials. Trials may use one of three methods: Larsen, Sharp and Sharp-van der Heijde.

Reproduced by kind permission of Elsevier Science Ltd. from van der Heijde et al. (1996)

space narrowing). There are specific ways of measuring changes identified in x-rays of the hands and feet. The metacarpophalangeal (MCP) joints of the hands and the metatarsophalangeal (MTP) joints of the feet are commonly affected by RA (Plant, 2001). The aim of examining x-rays is to determine the rate of disease progression. The small bones of the hands and feet are routinely assessed as they are commonly affected. However, other reasons for taking x-rays of these joints include the fact that a number of small joints can be seen with minimal radiation dose, it is relatively inexpensive and it is fairly easy to interpret the results. For research purposes, two of the most commonly used validated scoring systems for identifying very small degrees of difference in the rate of progression of the disease are the Sharp or the Larsen methods of assessing radiological progression. There are specific areas to assess and scrutinize in order to identify joint erosions and joint space narrowing (see Figure 7.6).

Conclusion

Evidence has shown that there remains a need for prompt treatment with DMARDs in order to reduce joint damage. It is likely that, for some time yet, DMARDs will remain the first treatment option for patients with inflammatory arthritis. However, it is disappointing to see that, despite encouraging results with DMARDs, radiographic progression continues for a significant proportion of patients (Pincus et al, 2002). This work has also been supported by others (Mulherin et al., 1996) who demonstrated joint erosions despite other clinical indicators (Ritchie Articular Index, haemoglobin and ESR) showing a significant benefit of treatment. (The Ritchie Articular Index is another way of examining joints to record a measure of disease activity, although it only scores tender joints. In clinical practice there has been a trend to use the 28-joint count DAS system, which measures both tender and swollen joints and probably takes less time to complete.) It is therefore important to note that reduction in radiographic progression is a key outcome for biologic therapies.

This chapter has identified current practice and highlighted the need to search for additional measures to evaluate benefits of treatment. As with all research work, increased evidence and knowledge will open new avenues for investigation. Anecdotally, clinical experience appears to highlight the overall improvement in the individual's sense of wellbeing and a reduction in fatigue following treatment with biologic therapies. There is a need to complement clinical indicators with outcomes that are patient-focused and attempt to capture global changes following treatment with biologic therapies.

There are also many important questions on the long-term safety and efficacy of treament with biologic therapies which should be answered in the next fews years. These include changes in the rate of joint replacements, emergency hospital admissions, access to additional healthcare resources, rate of infections and clarity about the theoretical risk of malignancies. It is clear to many that these therapies do provide significant benefit to many patients. It is therefore crucial that, as nurses, we increase our knowledge and expertise in the management of patients receiving biologic therapies to ensure that risk factors are reduced and a transparent process of care provides a framework that supports the patient in their decision making.

A detailed discussion on the responsibilities of practitioners caring for patients receiving biologic therapies is included in Chapter 8.

Chapter 8

Biologic therapies: practical aspects of care

Susan Oliver

Introduction

The immune process and the mechanism of action of biologic therapies have been discussed in Chapter 7. The aim of this chapter is to describe the aspects of care that should guide the preparation, assessment, administration and monitoring of patients receiving biologic therapies. It sets out:

- a framework for practice, including guidance documents necessary to adhere to nationally agreed policies
- guidance on aspects of safety and recognition of side effects related to biologic therapies
- how to develop standards of care for patients receiving biologic therapies
- how to identify resource implications
- how to recognize the patient's perspective.

The example of rheumatoid arthritis (RA) is used throughout the chapter to outline the practical issues in relation to care of patients receiving biologics. Some of the aspects of management outlined will have relevance for all chronic disease patients treated with biologics. Indeed, it is hoped that there will be initiatives for specialities to exchange clinical experiences and best practice. However, although there are some common factors in examining risks and benefits of treatment, nurses need also to be conversant with the validated measures necessary to observe changes in disease activity, research evidence and specific side-effect profiles related to the patient's condition. There may also be nationally agreed criteria and guidelines for management of specific disease areas.

Although these therapies are costly, they have the potential for significant improvement in the long-term outcomes for patients, so it is likely that there will be an increasing responsibility for healthcare professionals to demonstrate that they are assessing, administering and monitoring treatments using a structured, evidence-based approach. There are benefits in developing a standardized national approach to care. These include:

- an easy and transparent process ensuring equity of access
- enhancing the patient's understanding and therefore improving patient choice and the patient's journey
- demonstrating an evidence-based approach to care
- providing comprehensive and reproducible evidence on care in a clinical care setting
- guiding all healthcare professionals in the provision of care for patients receiving biologics (including outpatient nurses, day care nurses, multidisciplinary teams, clinical directors, drugs and therapeutic committees, clinical risk and clinical governance)
- providing a framework for the education of healthcare professionals
- highlighting the ongoing resource and developmental needs of the service.

Setting the framework

Developing evidence and standards of care

Over the past decade there has been an increasing trend to ensure that we provide the optimum in standards of care based on evidence-based research. Developing unified standards has the advantage that patients can have a clearer understanding of the decision-making processes and be active participants in discussions about the relative risks and benefits of specific treatment options. With the development of standards there is also a need to collect comprehensive evidence to assess the benefit of therapeutic interventions on patient outcomes. The principles of detailed evaluation have been applied to the introduction of the biologic therapies in RA.

British Society for Rheumatology

The British Society for Rheumatology (BSR) Working Party prepared guidelines for prescribing anti-tumour necrosis factor alpha (anti-TNFα) therapies (2000). Guidelines should not be considered a definitive document but a dynamic document that provides a framework for the practitioner to work with, guiding care, particularly in new areas of practice. Guidelines can often lag behind evolving issues in clinical practice and require regular review. The BSR guidelines (2000) have recently been amended to account for additional guidance on issue discussed in this chapter (e.g. tuberculosis (TB) and heart failure). At the time of writing the amendments had not been published but will be available on the BSR website (see Appendix 2).

The guidelines set out exclusion and inclusion criteria, as well as highlighting the clinical assessment process necessary to evaluate patients before starting treatment. Scotland has similar guidelines to the BSR (Table 8.1).

Table 8.1 Abbreviated British Society for Rheumatology guidelines for prescribing tumour necrosis factor alpha blockers with RA

Eligibility criteria

- Active RA - diagnosis should satisfy the American College of Rheumatology classification criteria for RA
- Active RA assessed using the 28 joint count disease activity score (DAS 28). Patient must have two DAS scores > 5.1 one month apart. A score of > 5.1 indicates high activity of disease
- Failure of at least two DMARDs, one of which should be methotrexate, at target doses following an adequate therapeutic trial (defined as treatment for at least 6 months, with at least 2 months at standard target dose - unless toxicity limits dose)

Exclusion criteria

Refer to summary of product characteristics (SPCs) for additional exclusion criteria:
- Women who are pregnant or breastfeeding
- Active infections including:
  - chronic leg ulcers
  - previous TB (if not previously treated)
  - septic arthritis of a native or prosthetic joint within the last 12 months
  - persistent or recurrent chest infections
  - indwelling urinary catheter
  - malignancy of pre-malignancy states, excluding basal cell carcinoma and malignancies diagnosed and treated more than 10 years previously (where probability of cure is very high)

Note: Women of childbearing potential and men receiving treatment should be advised to use an effective contraceptive.

Additional criteria:
SPC recommendations and proposed BSR amendments to guidelines

- Treatment should not be intiatied in patients with New York Heart Association grade 3 or 4 congestive cardiac failure (CCF)
- Treatment should be discontinued if CCF increases while on treatment
- Treatment should not be prescribed if history of demyelinating diseases

(BSR, 2000)

In the case of children and young adults with juvenile idiopathic arthritis (JIA), they should be cared for by specialist paediatric rheumatology services, and guidelines for assessment and management of etanercept have been prepared by the British Paediatric Rheumatology Group (BPRG, 2000). Similar groups have been formed in the USA and Europe to provide guidelines and support clinicians in the decision making for anti-TNFα treatments (Furst et al., 2002).

The BSR guidelines proved invaluable when the National Institute for Clinical Excellence (NICE) reviewed etanercept and infliximab in the treatment of RA and etanercept in JIA, as they provided a structured approach for the selection of patients. The BSR and BPRG guidelines were accepted as part of NICE guidance for infliximab and etanercept.

The National Institute for Clinical Excellence

NICE reviews medicines, devices, techniques and clinical management to identify 'best practice' (Rawlins, 2003). There is full discussion of the power and responsibilities of NICE in Chapters 1 and 10. The review process includes the wider aspects of 'effectiveness', including potential improvements to quality of life.

At the time of going to press two of the four licensed biologics (infliximab and etanercept) have been reviewed, and guidance on their use in the treatment of RA was published by NICE in March 2002 (NICE, 2002a). An additional guidance was issued at the same time for the use of etanercept for the treatment of JIA (NICE, 2002c). Anakinra has been reviewed by NICE for the treatment of RA and the final report is awaited.

NICE approval stipulates adherence to local and national audit to review practice. Table 8.2 outlines the key issues highlighted in NICE guidance for infliximab and etanercept for RA.

BSR Biologics Register

Ethical approval for a multicentre observational study was granted to the BSRBR. These data will provide national information as part of NICE implementation of biologics. The Biologic and New Drugs Register (BNDR) for children and young people collects similar data for the NICE guidance on the use of etanercept for JIA (NICE, 2002). There is adult representation on the BNDR to ensure linkage of data on young people to the adult Biologics Register (BR) at transition of young adults to the adult services.

The information collected by the adult register consists of patient

Table 8.2 NICE guidance on etanercept or infliximab for adults with rheumatoid arthritis

Patients should be eligible for treatment according to British Society for Rheumatology (BSR) guidelines (April, 2000)

- Patient should be prescribed etanercept or infliximab by a consultant rheumatologist. Choice of treatment should be decided taking into account different treatment schedules and patient preference
- All prescribing physicians should register the patient with the Biologics Register (www.arc.man.ac.uk). Additional information on dosage outcome and toxicity should be forwarded on a 6-monthly basis
- Treatment should be withdrawn in the event of severe drug-related toxicity or lack of response at 3 months
- Maintenance therapy should be at the lowest licensed dose compatible with clinical response
- Decisions about treatment continuing after 4 years of treatment will depend on the outcomes from the Biologics Register data

Implementation

- Review current practice in line with guidance
- Clinicians should audit compliance with guidance and BSR guidelines. Audit should include local monitoring protocols, the patient's knowledge of disease and the intended effect and potential adverse effects of treatment
- Prescribing physician responsible for registering patient on biologics register

Recommendations

- Etanercept or infliximab (infliximab only in combination with methotrexate) for adults with active RA who have not responded well to treatment with at least two DMARDs including methotrexate.
- Prescribed by a consultant rheumatologist
- Prescribed in accordance with BSR guidelines
- Patient consent needs to be sought for submission of relevant data to the Biologics Register. This information to be updated with the Biologics Register on a 6-monthly basis
- There is currently no evidence to support treatment after 4 years. Continuing treatment will need to be assessed on clinical assessment of disease control

diaries and questionnaires as well as a detailed clinical history. It is the responsibility of individual rheumatology units to inform the local research ethics committee of their participation in this multicentre observational study and the wish to collect data for the BSRBR register. Other European countries that have set up similar databases to review prospective data on biologic therapies include Germany, the Netherlands, Spain, Sweden and Norway.

Local units also need to collect data to audit their own adherence to NICE guidance. Data submitted to the BSRBR can be retrieved to inform local audit. The audit data will inform the NICE review process and provide essential evidence of data collected using a multicentre observational study approach over a five-year period.

A proposed electronic version of the BSRBR register has the potential to reduce clerical work and transfer the data electronically to the BSRBR, at the same time enabling the data to be stored electronically by the local rheumatology department. This will support both local and national data processing and reduce the practitioners' clerical workload.

The BSR guidelines started the process of setting a standard for care (BSR Working Party, 2000). The BSRBR and BNDR build on this framework, collecting observational data for all patients receiving these treatments to evaluate response and detection of adverse events. There is a need to evaluate the evolving evidence thoroughly, as the long-term effects of these drugs are, as yet, unknown. The data collection process is labour intensive but has the potential to have a significant impact on the overall provision of such treatments for patients in the future.

Although these new agents offer additional management options for the treatment of RA there remain some clear dilemmas for the clinician as to what is the best therapeutic regimen for the patient (Fries 2000). The evidence needs to be collated and relies on data collection prior to treatment and then should follow the patient's clinical progress throughout treatment. To review the BSRBR forms, refer to the website resources in Appendix 2.

The NICE review in 2005/2006 and subsequent decisions to continue to support the use of biologic therapies will have an impact on the future provision of biologics within the NHS. Although the strengths and weaknesses of this approach can be argued, if NICE do support an intervention in England and Wales, in principle the approved or recognized treatment should then be implemented within three months of this decision (NICE, 2001).

Implementing good practice

The Royal College of Nursing Rheumatology Nursing Forum (RCNRF) and members of the Arthritis and Musculoskeletal Alliance (ARMA) developed a guidance document providing comprehensive information to support practitioners (RCN, 2003a). The aim of the document was to provide a practical step-wise approach to the assessment, management and administration of biologic therapies for inflammatory arthritis. It provides practical guidance and information on all the key areas discussed in this chapter.

Practical aspects of care

The role of the nurse

The role of the nurse in caring for patients receiving targeted therapies is a significant one. The chronic disease patient is likely to have developed a trusting and supportive relationship with the team caring for them. This therapeutic relationship has evolved over time and various treatment interventions. In the past, when all traditional therapies were exhausted there were few options left, except perhaps drugs with significantly greater toxicity profiles, and many patients felt bereft of any hope of coping with their disease. Biologic therapies have provided new hope to those patients. The patient will be looking to the rheumatology team to support and advise them through what can seem a potentially difficult time in their disease. The nurse should:

- be competent in the screening and assessment process
- provide the patient with advice that is evidence based
- highlight the treatment options and relative risks and benefits of treatment
- support the patient in accessing appropriate information and opportunities to make an informed decision
- guide the patient and support healthcare professionals throughout the process of assessment, administration and monitoring
- ensure that the patient recognizes their responsibility in accepting treatment
- provide support for the patient if treatment is stopped
- provide information to the patient on how to access emergency care, details of their next treatment and the relevant follow-up care and monitoring.

Tables 8.3 and 8.4 provide guidance on a basic step-wise approach to assessing and administering treatment. However, for more detailed information refer to the RCN guidance document (2003a).

The patient's perspective

The patient should be an active participant in all aspects of their care. Holman and Lorig (2000) have highlighted improved satisfaction, concordance and continuity of care when patients are actively involved in decision making about their healthcare needs. This emphasis has also

Table 8.3 Preparation and screening of patients prior to anti-TNFα treatment

Prior to assessment

- Has the patient been counselled and fully informed about the risks and benefits of treatment and is this documented?
- Has the patient been given an opportunity to ask questions and had information backed up by literature?
- Has the patient's preference for treatment options been considered?

Assessment criteria

Ensure that the patient is eligible for treatment based on BSR guidelines for two DMARDs* at target dosage.

- 28 tender and swollen joint counts, patient global assessment of disease activity
- Bloods for FBC*, ESR*, CRP*
- Early morning stiffness
- Additional documented measures of ongoing disease activity (e.g. Health Assessment Questionnaire for Biologics Register)
- Exclusion of active infection (e.g. septic arthritis) or infections of any prosthesis in last 12 months (document number of prosthesis)
- Exclusion of chronic infections (e.g. leg ulcers) or persistent infections
- Patients screened for previous tuberculosis contacts or risk of TB*
- If a patient has had a chest x-ray within the last 6 months, review the x-ray with pre-scribing physician. If the patient has not had an chest x-ray within the last 6 months, review with prescribing physician for consideration
- Malignancy (exclude if treatment within the last 10 years and chance of cure very high) or pre-malignancy, e.g. basal cell carcinoma
- Discuss any personal or family history of demyelinating disease with prescribing physician
- Data advises caution in the use of anti-TNFα treatments in moderate to severe heart failure
- If patient is eligible following the above assessment a Disease Activity Score (DAS) should be calculated
- Patients are eligible if they have a DAS score higher than 5.1 measured at two time points one month apart
- The effectiveness of treatment will then be assessed at each infusion and reviewed around the time of the fourth infusion with the prescribing physician
- Patients are expected to achieve at least a DAS score reduction of < 3.2 or improve by > 1.2 at the 3-month assessment point

*CRP: C-Reactive Protein   DMARD: Disease Modifying Anti-Rheumatic Drugs
ESR: Erythrocyte Sedimentation Rate   FBC: Full Blood Count   TB: Tuberculosis

been supported in the Department of Health documents *The Expert Patient* (DoH, 2001b) and *Good Practice in Consent: implementation guide* (DoH, 2001d).

The nurse must have a good understanding of the patient's perceptions and any psychological issues that may affect individual views of treatment

Table 8.4 Before starting anti-TNFα treatment

- Ensure that informed consent has been obtained from the patient and they fulfil criteria for treatment
- Patients should not be breastfeeding, considering conception or be pregnant. An effective method of contraceptive should be used
- Patient should have been thoroughly screened for any infections or changes in general health (e.g. breathlessness, cough or neurological signs)
- DAS score assessed
- Review pre-infusion bloods. Bloods for FBC and ESR
- Temperature, blood pressure, pulse recorded
- Ensure patient is eligible for treatment prior to preparing anti-TNFα for administration
- For subcutaneous therapies – plan and prepare adequate training time to teach patient self-administration of subcutaneous injection
- Check dosage calculated according to patient's weight (for infliximab)
- Ensure administration of infusions (infliximab) is via a low protein-binding filter using a infusion pump
- If patient has had an infusion reaction at previous administration, discuss with prescribing physician the option of antihistamine and paracetamol prior to administration of the infusion

As with any other infusion emergency resuscitation equipment should be readily available in case of anaphylaxis

For infusions

- Review all pre-treatment observations and blood results before cannulation
- Administration of prophylactic treatment if required.
- Baseline and half-hourly observations during the infusion

Following administration of treatment

- Ensure that the patient is stable. Infliximab infusions – observe patient for 1-2 hours post-infusion
- Provide contact numbers for patients. Ensure that the patient has a patient alert card identifying their last dose administered
- Agree a telephone review contact and next treatment date
- Advise patient to seek early medical advice if aware of raised temperatures of other signs of early infection
- If patient has been adequately trained in self-administration of subcutaneous injection techniques, ensure that all equipment is available and the patient is confident and competent
- Arrange next blood monitoring review/telephone review

Cautions and unwanted side effects

- Injection site or infusion reactions are the commonest side effects
- Treatment should be stopped if serious infection, allergic reactions, pancytopenia or aplastic anaemia occurs
- Be vigilant for any signs of infection or possible TB
- Live vaccines must be avoided
- Treatment with anti-TNFα has been associated with demyelinating diseases (e.g. multiple sclerosis)
- Caution in patients with heart failure or worsening symptoms following treatment failure

Key DAS: Disease Activity Score   ESR: Erythrocyte Sedimentation Rate
FBC: Full Blood Count   TB: Tuberculosis

options (e.g. confidence, fear, expectations, acceptance of lack of efficacy and side effects). The level of support that nurses and other members of the team provide can have a significant impact on the patient's confidence and ability to cope (Newbold, 1996; Carter et al., 2003). Patient concordance has also been linked to improved communication and the quality of interactions between the patient and healthcare professionals (Cameron, 1996).

Individuals may experience a sense of euphoria with heightened expectations and hopes that are invested in treatment, particularly when all other treatments have failed. These expectations are often met (for about 70% of patients). However, evidence suggests that those who fail the recognized DAS criteria for benefit of treatment may still demonstrate benefit in the form of reductions in expected joint erosions on x-ray (Lipsky et al, 2000). When patients stop treatment, having tried a range of biologic therapies, there are currently no easy options for them to return to. A significant and essential aspect of providing care for patients receiving biologic therapies is that of supporting those who fail due to either recurrent serious infections or failure to demonstrate the necessary benefit from treatment. The specialist skills of all the team will need to be deployed to support the patient (physically and psychologically) in finding the optimum way to manage their disease without biologic therapies.

Equally important is that the patient is aware of the different forms of biologic therapies and their route of administration. The patient should be carefully assessed and options discussed with them to ensure (where appropriate) that the patient's preference in choice and route of administration is considered. The deciding factors that inform a patient's decision or opinion on which therapy would be most appropriate for them can sometimes be surprising and cannot be predicted. For example:

- A young single parent may :
  - choose intravenous therapy to avoid having syringes and medical equipment around the house
  - not wish to be seen as 'sick' and receiving treatment in hospital
  - need the reassurance of regular contact while having an infusion with nursing and medical staff reviewing care.

- A patient with long-standing disease with a fear of needles may:
  - choose subcutaneous administration to beat their fears and gain a sense of 'control'
  - prefer not to 'think about it' and wish to have an infusion
  - not want to ask their partner for aid in subcutaneous administration (independence, poor relationships).

There are additional factors that healthcare professionals need to consider and discuss with the patient:

- There may be issues of concordance with treatment regimens and monitoring that will need to be discussed to decide on the most appropriate treatment.
- The patient may prefer the convenience of subcutaneous administration, avoiding the need for hospital visits.
- A home environment that is not conducive to home administration of treatment.
- Social and psychological factors that may need to be considered.
- Poor venous access.
- Risk factors that may necessitate specific choices of treatment (e.g. patient with multiple sclerosis).

Preparing the patient

Treatment options

The patient must have the opportunity to make a true informed decision on whether to accept or refuse any treatment offered (Dimond, 2002). The role in preparing patients for targeted therapies may start when the disease fails to be adequately controlled and traditional disease-modifying anti-rheumatic drugs (DMARDs) have been ineffective.

The patient should be aware of the treatment criteria for biologics and be informed about the options available to them in their decision making. This may help to clarify why the patient has not yet been considered for treatment, reassure the patient on the other aspects of care or treatment that are available to them, and balance heightened and perhaps unrealistic expectations. There should be no mystery about why some patients are being treated with 'new' drugs and others are not.

Patients undergoing significant crises with an uncertain future will need to be supported and counselled carefully about the relative risks and benefits. Information should be provided in all formats, enabling the patient to reflect on the options and discuss them with their relatives or close friends. The patient should then be offered a further opportunity to ask questions and review their decision. Complex research evidence and relative risks and benefits of treatment need to be conveyed in different ways according to the patient's specific wishes (for example, coping styles) and their ability to assimilate the knowledge (Hill, 1998). A more in-depth discussion on the patient issues related to treatment is included in Chapter 4.

However, there are a number of key issues that the patient should be aware of:

- They should understand the current criteria for treatment and choice of therapies.
- The clarity of the screening process and rationale behind thorough and regular assessments.
- The should receive information about the various treatment options and consideration should be taken of their personal history and preferences.
- The risks and benefits of treatment (this should be discussed in the context of the patient's own clinical history).
- The patient's responsibility in receiving treatment (e.g. regular attendance for reviews and assessments, blood monitoring, prompt treatment of infections).
- The rationale behind data for BSR, BR and NICE guidance.
- The reasons why treatment may be stopped.
- The support available through the hospital, primary care teams and patient groups.
- The use of the patient alert card and helpline services.
- The patient should be encouraged to review/discuss any of the above information by requesting a further appointment.

The assessment process

The patient receiving targeted therapies will have to accept a rigorous assessment process. During the nursing assessment and screening processes there will be opportunities to ensure that the individual has been well informed about the treatment and has had an opportunity to review the literature and ask questions about their treatment. The thorough screening process reinforces the importance of monitoring for infections.

For some, the detailed assessment and review processes can be reassuring, but for others they will raise anxieties. The patient must be encouraged to recognize that they will need to invest in time, either receiving treatment or learning to administer their own treatment. This involves a degree of commitment for the patient, including attending regularly for clinical reviews and blood monitoring. The assessment process includes:

- Identification of patients eligible for treatment according to BSR criteria (see Table 8.1).
- Preparation of BSRBR data and patient consent forms.
- Screening process that includes a medical assessment, clinical history (physical and mental health), blood monitoring and chest x-ray.
- Active participation of the patient in all aspects of the decision making, including specialist education and written information on potential risks and benefits of treatment. This must include criteria for commencing and stopping treatment

- Ensuring that the patient consents to treatment and recognizes their responsibilities in receiving treatments and that there is appropriate documentation of these discussions.
- Co-prescribing of methotrexate according to the SPC for some biologic therapies.
- Assessment of appropriate route of administration based on the patient's views and functional ability, and optimum treatment based on medical and social history.
- Documentation and administrative work in preparing for subcutaneous administration or day case admission for treatment.
- Planned management of patients who fail the eligibility criteria or elect not to receive biologic therapies.

See Chapter 7 for an outline of characteristics of biologic treatments available for RA (for detailed information on the licensed therapies refer to the SPC sheets available at www.medicines.org.uk).

Understanding the risks and benefits of treatment

Chapter 7 outlines the benefits of biologic therapies to patients. Patients who are currently assessed and eligible for treatment in the UK must fail at least two standard DMARDs at target dosages, one of which must be methotrexate. They must also fulfil the rigorous inclusion criteria. This often means that patients receiving biologics have complex disease and are likely to have joint damage (and possibly joint replacements). Patients may also be immunocompromised following long-term treatment with disease-modifying drugs and possibly steroid treatment.

Post-marketing surveillance (PMS) and research evidence continue to inform care. In particular, following the introduction of biologic therapies into routine clinical practice, Moots et al. (2003) have emphasized the importance of clinical screening to ensure that the patient is assessed and screened before commencing treatment.

Biologics: risks and benefits

When considering the risks of treatment, it is important to take account of the complex chronic disease status of patients currently receiving biologic therapies. There are a number of common characteristics in terms of safety data that need to be discussed:

- susceptibility to infections, including TB

- theoretical risk of malignancy for anti-TNFα therapies
- caution in their use by patients with moderate-to-severe cardiac failure
- demyelinating diseases
- abnormal blood results
- sensitivity reactions
- co-prescribing DMARDs.

Susceptibility to infections

The mechanism of action of biologic therapies is to 'block or disarm' cytokines that would usually instigate an inflammatory response. Equally, complex chronic disease patients are at an increased risk of opportunistic infections. The most common infections, including TB, are set out in Table 8.5.

Table 8.5 Infections

Infection	Biologic therapy	Details	Comments
Tuberculosis (TB)	All biologic therapies	Adalimumab Etanercept Infliximab Anakinra	• Deaths have occurred from TB • High prevalence of TB internationally in normal (e.g. non-rheumatoid arthritis) population • Ensure thorough screening. Refer to RCN guidance (2003) • Post-marketing surveillance reiterated screening process • One case of TB reported with anakinra (Medical Information, Amgen, June, 2003).
Injection site reactions (ISR) All classified as transient mild to moderate infusion reactions	Subcutaneous therapies: adalimumab/ anakinra /etanercept	Anakinra, adalimumab and etanercept describe ISRs as very common (> 10%)	• Mild or moderate ISRs are common but normally resolve without treatment • Occasionally may require topical treatment to reduce discomfort (hydrocortisone cream)
Respiratory tract infections and other opportunistic infections Includes mild to moderate infections	All therapies	Adalimumab common > 5%; anakinra common 1-10%; etanercept very common > 10%; infliximab common < 10%	• Deaths have occurred from opportunistic infections • Ensure patient is aware of the need to report infections and obtain prompt treatment • Defer treatment if serious infections • Review with prescribing physician if infections are suspected

Sources: Data from Summary of Product Characteristics, Abbott, Amgen, Schering Plough and Wyeth (2003) Medical Information Departments of Abbott, Amgen; Strand 2002.

The essential 'safety net' is that of ensuring that the patient accepts and understands the need to report any potential infection promptly. This can occasionally be a problem when patients feel significantly better as a result of treatment and may fail to recall the need to seek treatment; equally they may be anxious about treatment being stopped as a result of an infection.

Tuberculosis

One-third of the total world population is infected with TB (Kaufmann, 2002). However, fewer than 10% will ever develop the disease, although the pathogen is not always eradicated but contained in discrete lesions (Kaufmann, 2002). The immune system is normally effective in containing the pathogen, although it may fail to eradicate it. The increasing incidence of TB internationally highlights the need to ensure that any possible TB contact or history of TB should be taken seriously.

Deaths as a result of TB infection have been associated with all anti-TNFα treatments internationally. The time to presentation of Mycobacterium TB (M.TB) differs significantly with a mean time of offset of 11.2 months with etanercept, wheres 97% of infliximab-treated patients developed M.TB within seven months (Keystone, 2003). In the light of the evidence that suggests that there is a risk of TB reactivation following treatment with biologic therapies, the British Thoracic Society Working Party is preparing guidance for screening of patients receiving biologics and treatment that they may require if a positive test for TB is reported. This includes the risks related to the side effects associated with anti-tuberculosis treatment, which are not insignificant (Joint Tuberculosis Committee of the British Thoracic Society, 2003).

Patients born before 1942 will not have had the benefit of the TB immunization programmes in the UK. The area of immunization and appropriate methods of diagnosing TB are complex and require detailed analysis of clinical history, investigations and thorough review of chest x-rays. For a detailed discussion, refer to the RCN guidance document (2003a).

Theoretical risk of malignancy

As discussed in Chapter 7, anti-TNFα has a role in the destruction of pre-malignant cells. There is therefore a theoretical risk of malignancy by blocking the cytokine TNFα. However, this theoretical risk to date has not been supported by the PMS. Patients with active RA have a marginally increased risk of malignancy, partly due to the disease process but also as a result of drug therapies (Abu-Shakra et al., 2001). The statistics to date show that the expected rate of malignancies has not changed in those patients receiving biologics. The role of the BSRBR will include the scrutiny of patient outcomes related to malignancies.

Heart failure

PMS data from Schering Plough (infliximab) have highlighted a risk to patients with moderate or severe heart failure (New York Heart Association III or IV). It should be used with caution in patients who have mild heart failure and should be discontinued if their heart failure worsens (Schering Plough, 2003). The same guidance should be applied to other anti-TNFα therapies until evidence is available to the contrary. PMS and SPCs for etanercept support this guidance (Schering Plough, 2003; Wyeth, 2003).

Demyelinating disease

It has been shown that anti-TNFα does not provide clinical benefit to patients with multiple sclerosis (MS) and in fact may exacerbate the disease (Robinson et al., 2001). It is therefore essential to ensure that patients with a history of demyelinating disease are excluded from treatment. A prescribing physician should review patients who develop signs or symptoms suggestive of a neurological problem. The causal relationship between anti-TNFα treatments and MS remains unclear.

Blood monitoring

Blood and lymphatic disorders have been documented with all of the biologic therapies. However, many patients may also be co-prescribed DMARDs, steroids and anti-inflammatories. It is therefore good clinical practice to review the patient's blood results regularly. Scrutiny of blood results should include checking for elevated white cell counts, as well as measuring inflammatory markers for DAS assessments.

For treatments that require the co-prescribing of methotrexate, regular blood monitoring is usually undertaken once a month when established on treatment (RCN, 2003a). It is good practice to ensure that individuals receiving treatment by infusion have a blood result available in the week preceding the infusion. Details of blood disorders are documented in Table 8.6.

Blood monitoring: antibodies to treatment

With all biologic therapies, patients with positive antibodies (e.g. antibodies to adalimumab, anakinra, infliximab or etanercept) have been

Table 8.6 Blood-related disorders in treatment with biologic therapies

Treatment	Blood disorder	Results seen	Comments
Adalimumab* (Weinblatt et al., 2003) Ref: FDA 2002	No documented blood disorders related to drug-related toxicity ANA Anti-dsDNA antibodies	Positive ANA and dsDNA results seen (some in placebo group)	One case of lupus-like syndrome (from a population of 2334 patients) developed – recovered on cessation of treatment (Medical Information, Abbott, January 2003)
Anakinra (Bresnihan et al., 1998; Bresnihan, 2000)	Common	Neutropenia	Treatment should not be initiated if neutrophil count is low. Review with prescribing physician
		No cases of positive ANA/dsDNA in clinical trials	One case of lupus-like syndrome in PMS* (Medical Information, Amgen, June 2003)
Etanercept	Uncommon	Thrombocytopenia	Caution in patients with a history of blood dyscrasias
	Rare	Anaemia, leukopenia, pancytopenia	
	Very rare	Aplastic anaemia ANA and dsDNA antibodies. Positive ANA and dsDNA results seen	No cases of lupus-like syndromes
Infliximab	Uncommon	Anaemia, leukopenia, lymphadenopathy, neutropenia, thrombocytopenia	
	Rare	pancytopenia	
	Uncommon	ANA and dsDNA antibodies. Positive ANA and dsDNA results seen	Rare cases of clinical signs of lupus-like syndromes. Anti-dsDNA reverts to normal on cessation of treatment

Key ANA: Anti-Nuclear Antibody   dsDNA: Double Stranded DNA   FDA: Federal Drug Administration
*No post-marketing data. Information taken from Adalimumab Medicines Information Pack, Abbott Laboratories (2003) and Medicines Information Department, Abbott Laboratories (unpublished). Information provided in spring 2003. At the time of writing, this information reflected information obtained from either Medical Information Departments of the pharmaceutical company or documented information in the Summary of Product Characteristics (accessed on www.emc.vhn.net in spring 2003; new website address www.medicines.org.uk)

identified. The clinical significance of these antibodies is not yet fully understood, although it is thought that they might affect the patient therapeutic response to treatment.

It has also been reported that some patients receiving biologic therapies become positive for anti-nuclear antibodies (ANAs) and anti-double stranded DNA. It is useful to ensure that a baseline blood test is taken and reviewed if patients develop symptoms of lupus-like symptoms. The occurrence of lupus-like syndromes is very rare and usually resolves when treatment is stopped.

Sensitivity reactions

The most common sensitivity reactions to treatment are injection site reactions with subcutaneous injections and mild infusion reactions with infliximab. The infusion reactions are more likely in the first few infusions, although they can present at any time. They usually resolve with little or no treatment. However, as biologic therapies are derived from proteins, occasionally moderate to severe reactions can occur.

As with any protein-derived intravenous therapy there is always the potential risk of anaphylactic shock. As part of normal clinical practice in administering any treatment, nurses should ensure that they are competent in caring for patients receiving treatment and are aware of local trust policies to treat moderate to severe reactions.

Some units have chosen to administer prophylactic treatment (such as paracetamol and antihistamine) prior to infusion to patients who have previously had a mild infusion reaction. A small study on Crohn's disease patients by Cheifetz et al. (2001) suggests that prophylaxis may be effective in reducing the risk of subsequent reactions.

The RCN (2003a) document provides a step-wise approach to the care of patients receiving treatment and also outlines relevant documents to access and guidelines that can be adapted to adhere to local practice.

Co-prescribing DMARDs

Some biologic therapies require additional co-prescribing of methotrexate or another DMARD. This can present a problem, as the DMARD may have already been tried, and problems with tolerance or side effects necessitate cessation of treatment. Recently there has been an increasing use of parental methotrexate to improve absorption and tolerance, particularly when higher dosages are administered (up to 25mg weekly). Although there is no definitive guidance on using alternative DMARDs, some prescribing physicians have elected to prescribe a DMARD that does not adhere to the licensed indication for the biologic agent (e.g. infliximab SPC states co-prescribing with methotrexate). A research trial examining a small group of RA patients (*n* = 20) receiving infliximab and leflunomide demonstrated benefits to treatment, but the adverse events were high, with 55% of patients having to withdraw due to side effects (Kiely and Johnson, 2002).

Reporting adverse events

Although new therapies have undergone rigorous research in clinical trials, new and sometimes very relevant clinical adverse events can evolve over time. There are a number of reasons for this. In research studies, patients are rigorously screened and have to pass very clear inclusion and exclusion criteria. In clinical care, this is not always the case, therefore patients may have other complex disease processes that may cause additional problems, for example the development of a drug interaction between the biologic therapy and another prescribed treatment.

Nurses should be aware of these issues and the fact that, once a new drug is licensed, less 'controlled' groups of patients will be receiving treatment. It is therefore normal practice for the use of an early warning system to identify to pharmaceutical companies and ultimately practitioners any potential new problems with a newly licensed drug. It is for these reasons that PMS should be collected. In the UK, this is an alert 'yellow card' system used by the Medicines Control Agency.

If any side effects are significant and possibly related to the administration of a drug, the prescribing physician should document this using an alert card system. This reporting system has been officially authorized for the use of nurses as well as prescribing physicians (Medicines Control Agency, 2002). The alert/yellow card can be found in the appendix of the *British National Formulary*.

Defining the resource implications

It can be seen that these biologic therapies have implications for the provision of care for patients receiving them. Although NICE (2002a) supported the treatment of infliximab and etanercept, it failed to recognize the resource implications for nurses. It now rests with many units, and particularly senior nurses, to identify ways of providing an adequate support system to counsel, assess and if not administer treatment, and provide specialist support to day units or wards.

Implementing a new service provision requires a collaborative approach between all the healthcare professionals involved in the care of patients with RA. A review of the assessment process, appropriate documentation, and responsibility of counselling and preparing the patient for treatment all need to be clarified. As discussed, vigilance in all aspects of care is essential. In some units, this will be carried out by the prescribing consultant; in others the nurses will undertake a significant proportion of this work.

The nurse may need to review the local guidelines or protocols for teaching patients to self-administer subcutaneous injections if the unit decides not to use pharmaceutical nursing support to train patients. If the patient is to receive regular infusions, the availability of day care facilities or inpatient beds may need to be reviewed as well as nursing expertise in intravenous administration and management. Whatever therapy the patient is receiving, the important aspect is that of regular assessment and reviews to ensure that the treatment is effective and that there are no monitoring or care issues.

The shortfall in the provision of specialist expertise and resources to administer treatments has been recognized by pharmaceutical companies, and various packages of support have been developed to aid in the care of patients receiving biologic therapies.

Nurses need to ensure that they are looking at the strategic development of their service, ensuring not only that care can be provided in the short term, but that they are able to plan for future service provision. To do this, a structured framework needs to be set out, identifying the competencies required as well as resource implications in delivery care (Table 8.7). There are a number of options that can be considered initially:

- Prepare a business proposal to gain additional funding and resources (see Chapter 2).
- Work in new ways to enhance knowledge and provide additional non-specialist support (e.g. train day unit nurses in screening and assessment prior to administration of biologic therapies).
- Identify with management ways of optimizing funds allocated for administration of biologics. This may enable additional nursing or resources to be generated to ensure that patients have treatment safely administered.

The patient will expect competent practitioners to manage their care. The lead practitioner as well as the individual practitioners will need to evaluate their own competencies as well as facilities and expertise appropriate to administering care (Nursing and Midwifery Council, 2002c)

The key aspects of service provision to be reviewed are:

- competencies: review of training and educational needs
- cascading knowledge and skills
- facilities and resources: environment and facilities available for administration and support
- infrastructure: departments required to support the administration and care of patients – pharmacy, day unit facilities, outpatient clinics, helpline

Table 8.7 Service development planning

Screening	Resource implication	Practitioner	Competencies
Screening and assessment	Clinic and nursing time	Specialist skills	Joint assessment skills DMARD knowledge BSR/Biologics Register/NICE guidelines/RCN guidelines
Counselling	Clinic and nursing time	Specialist skills	Evidence-based research on DMARDs and biologics Psychological and social issues related to RA
Treatment administration	Protocols/clinic/ nursing Facilities/resources	Specialist skills	Experience in preparing protocols Expertise in supervisory role/managing supporting role Ability to negotiate with management
Training of patients and staff	Visiting/ administration Documentation	Non-specialist but supported by specialist skills	Intravenous and/or subcutaneous expertise and knowledge of drug interactions/adverse events
Administration and follow-up	Telephone reviews/monitoring Planning resources Pharmacy liaison	Specialist skills Secretarial/ clerical	Communication and liaison with specialist team Expertise in helpline support and resources required
Service development and access to resources/day care facilities	Business case proposals/education and training	Specialist skills Multidisciplinary support	Knowledge of disease process and management Experience in teamwork and NHS care Managerial skills and specialist knowledge In-depth grasp of research evidence

- patient needs in relation to the administration of targeted therapies
- documentation, e.g. Biologics Register, policies, guidelines.

Conclusions

For many individuals with RA, their difficulties are compounded by other chronic conditions or complexities as a result of their aggressive disease. The expertise in managing individuals with RA relies not only on a sound knowledge of the disease and the disease process, but also on a good foundation in chronic disease management, observing for side effects of treatment, infection or an increase in disease activity. There is a need for nurses to respond promptly in a knowledgeable way in order to improve patient care, and this often involves taking on new skills to cope with new patient problems (Hunt and Wainwright, 1994).

The development of nurse-led clinics has helped patients with rheumatological conditions to cope with many of these difficulties. Hill et al. (1994, 2003a) have demonstrated the effectiveness and safety of nurse clinics in rheumatology. Nurses and practitioners have demonstrated their ability to develop services based on patient need. Biologic therapies present new challenges for healthcare resources, however there are significant potential benefits to the patient and the provision of care if the planning and development of services is managed effectively.

There are opportunities and challenges for the development of new and innovative ways of working to develop a service that can ensure that patients have equity of access to treatment. The extent to which nurses will need or wish to extend their practice will vary depending on the needs of the patient group and those of the individual units.

An essential aspect of the nurse's role is that of ensuring that those patients who wish to receive treatment have given true informed consent and have had an opportunity to discuss any concerns they have. Equally, nurses must demonstrate expertise in managing patients with this complex chronic disease. Patients need to be appropriately assessed, monitored and managed while receiving these new treatments. The safety and efficacy of the drug requires regular assessment of disease activity and good communication with the patient. In many cases, the rheumatology nurse helpline services have proved invaluable in ensuring that contact is effectively maintained (see Chapter 3).

If a clear framework is set out it will help to identify resource implications and individual practitioner's responsibilities. The long-term funding for targeted therapies in the NHS will rely on good audit trails and data collection via the Biologics Register. Currently, the NICE guidance and evidence supports treatment for up to four years. Nurses have a key role in ensuring the safety of patients, adherence to NICE guidance and ultimately the future equitable provision of biologic therapies.

If the long-term safety and efficacy of these drugs can be demonstrated it heralds an exciting development in the treatment and care of patients with RA. There are a wide range of potential benefits to patients, including: reduction in joint destruction and the subsequent need for joint replacements, improvements in functional ability and the resulting social consequences of patients being able to take a more active part in society.

Chapter 9

Joint injections

Sarah Ryan

Introduction

The number of nurses and other health professionals within rheumatology who are involved in extended roles is increasing (Carr, 2002). Role extension refers to nurses carrying out tasks not included in their normal training for registration. These tasks are mainly acute medical interventions that are normally carried out by doctors (Wright, 1995). Aspects of practice that can regarded as examples of role extension include managing caseloads, ordering and interpreting diagnostic investigations, prescribing treatments, making and receiving referrals from other specialities, and joint injections. Intra-articular (IA) steroid injections were introduced into rheumatological practice by Hollander in the 1950s (Hollander et al., 1951) and are now the most frequently performed procedure, taking place in 12% of all consultations (Bamji et al., 1990).

One of the main objectives of nursing practice is to provide comprehensive, holistic care to improve patient outcomes. Role extension can be utilized to achieve this objective. This chapter focuses on two main areas: the professional and legal aspects that underpin nursing practice, and the evidence base supporting joint aspirations and injections.

The information provided in this chapter should enable the reader to:

- discuss the professional and legal issues surrounding the administration of IA injections
- explain the evidence for using IA corticosteroids in nursing practice
- describe the contraindications and potential complications of IA injections
- educate and support a patient having a joint injection.

Professional and legal issues

Role development

The 1990s saw a growth in the number of nurses conducting assessment clinics for patients with inflammatory arthritis. As the nurses' knowledge and skills increased, the debate over whether they should be able to give IA injections arose. Traditionally, doctors have given IA injections, but as nurses became more involved in the holistic care management of patients it appeared a natural step to develop their skills to be able to perform this procedure. Before this development, a nurse reviewing a patient's care may have had to interrupt the therapeutic consultation to find a medical colleague to perform an aspiration and injection of a joint that they assessed as requiring this procedure. The patient would then have had to wait for a doctor to be free. It seemed more beneficial to the patient's needs if the nurse who was providing a comprehensive evaluation of the patient's physical, psychological and social needs could develop the knowledge and skills in examination and injection to add to the holistic care already being provided. Other drivers that have influenced this aspect of role development include:

- the introduction of *The Scope of Professional Practice* (UKCC, 1992), which provided a framework for nurses to develop their skills in accordance with patients' needs and enabled the profession to make its own decisions and take responsibility for its actions
- the reduction in junior doctors' hours and the political emphasis on the need to reduce waiting lists
- the continued development of nursing roles to improve patient care as portrayed in the Chief Nursing Officer's ten key roles (see Appendix 1).

Table 9.1 shows the clinical components of the rheumatology nurse's role.

Professional and legal issues

Prior to *The Scope of Professional Practice* (UKCC, 1992) there was no formalized structure for nurses carrying out an extended role such as cannulation or venepuncture. Each trust devised its own system of training, which usually involved a nurse observing how a task was carried out, undergoing a period of supervised practice and then being given a certificate to state that they were competent in this procedure.

The system had a number of limitations (RCN Survey, 1990):

- Nurses developed only technical skills without the appropriate wider knowledge base.

Table 9.1 The clinical role components of rheumatology nurses

Role	Percentage of nurses who routinely perform the role
Give information and advice to patients	82
Read/record blood results	73
Give information and advice to relatives	71
Refer to other health professionals	58
Provide counselling for patients	54
Run drug-monitoring clinics	53
Order clinical investigations	52
Joint injections	12

Source: Carr (2001)

- There was no ongoing assessment of competence once the certificate had been issued.
- There was no formal recognition of training between trusts so a nurse who moved trusts would have to undergo the same training again.

In 1992, the government and the UKCC acknowledged the limitation of extended role training and practice and introduced *The Scope of Professional Practice* (1992). The guiding principles are shown in Table 9.2.

The principles set out in *The Scope of Professional Practice* can be applied to the scenario of a nurse administering IA injections. This practice is directed towards meeting the needs of a patient with an effusion related to the exacerbation of their rheumatoid arthritis (RA), and there is evidence to support the efficacy of this practice (Dorman and Ravin, 1991). The Scope clearly states that nurses should not just have the skills to perform IA injections but must have the appropriate knowledge base to support decision making and demonstrate competency in this area of practice. If the nurse is developing practice by taking on new skills, any

Table 9.2 The Scope of Professional Practice

Each registered nurse must:

- Be satisfied that each area of practice is directed to meeting the needs and serving the interests of the patients
- Endeavour always to achieve, maintain and develop knowledge, skills and competence to respond to these needs and interest
- Acknowledge any limitations of knowledge and skills
- Avoid any inappropriate delegation

delegation of other areas of the workload must be done appropriately, with colleagues having the knowledge and skills to take on new areas of practice.

Accountability

Pennels (1997) defines accountability as the requirement for each nurse to be responsible and answerable for the outcome of his or her professional actions (see Table 9.3). The code of professional conduct (NMC, 2002) alludes to all these areas because it states that as a registered nurse you must:

- protect and support the health of individual patients and clients
- protect and support the health of the wider community
- act in such a way that justifies the trust and confidence the public have in you
- uphold and enhance the good reputation of the professions.

Table 9.3 Accountability

The nurse is accountable to:

- the public – through criminal law
- the employer – through contract law
- the patient – through a legal duty to care and through civil law
- the profession through the Nursing and Midwifery Council (NMC).

Employer liability

There are two types of liability:

- Direct liability, e.g. the hospital is held responsible for an outbreak of food poisoning.
- Vicarious or indirect liability – the employer, e.g. the trust, is responsible for the faults or civil wrongs of others, provided that the employee:
  - is on duty at the time of the wrong
  - is working within the parameters of their job description and contract
  - adheres to policies, procedures, guidelines and protocols.

In theory (although it is unlikely to occur in practice), an employer could waive the right to cover the employee if these conditions are not adhered to. The job description should be a dynamic tool accurately reflecting the role that the individual is engaged in. In the case of a nurse who has undergone training and developed the knowledge and skills to be competent in the practice of IA injections, the job description should reflect this new aspect of practice.

The employer will need to approve any enhancement of the nurse's role, provide the relevant education and training, and ratify the guidelines and/or patient group directions under which the nurse will work through the appropriate trust processes (e.g. ratification by the local drugs and therapeutics committee or clinical governance group).

Civil law affecting nursing practice

The two main areas of civil law relevant to the changing roles of nurses are negligence and battery (Dowling et al., 1996). Negligence has to be proved on three accounts.

1 A nurse owed a duty of care to a patient.
2 There has been a breach of that duty.
3 As a result of that breach the patient has suffered damage.

A nurse who has been deemed competent to carry out joint injections is expected to use reasonable care and skills in the application of the injection. If the nurse deviates from the ratified guidelines for this procedure and as a result the patient suffers an unfavourable reaction, e.g. a pneumothorax following a shoulder injection, the patient may take legal action for negligence. Negligence charges can arise from the act, omission or inappropriate delegation, e.g. a nurse asking a colleague who has not been formally assessed as being competent to perform the injection. Ignorance of guidelines, policies and protocols can also lead to a charge of negligence

The standard of care

The court determines what would have been a reasonable action in a particular set of circumstances through the application of the Bolam test (*Bolam v Friern Hospital Management Committee* 1957):

> the test is the standard of the ordinary skilled man exercising and professing to have that special skill. A man need not possess the highest expert skill at the risk of being found negligent . . . it is sufficient if he exercises the ordinary skills of an ordinary man exercising that particular art.

If a negligence charge is brought against a nurse performing joint injections, the court would compare the circumstances with another nurse competent in this activity. The court would consider whether the actions of the nurse against whom the charges have been brought would have been reasonable to expect from a nurse professing to be competent in this activity.

The legal system is now moving towards utilizing clinical guidelines as a benchmark, with best practice rather than reasonable practice being the expected norm.

Consent

The method of consent most frequently obtained is verbal consent, which should be clearly elicited from the patient and recorded in the patient's documentation. There is considerable discussion within the profession as to whether verbal consent should be replaced by written consent for all invasive procedures. Patient consent and relevant documentation relating to consent have been published in a reference document (DoH, 2001d).

The following aspects must be considered when preparing a patient to consent for an IA injection:

- Nurses are accountable for ensuring that the patient has given consent for any treatment that they are giving (NMC, 2002b).
- Consent should be obtained only after the nurse has given the patient adequate information in order for him or her to make a meaningful decision (Table 9.4).
- The patient has the capacity to obtain and comprehend information and make an informed decision about the proposed intervention.
- If the nurse is performing the procedure, he or she should be the one to obtain the consent. It would be unacceptable practice for the doctor to obtain consent and then the practice to be carried out by the nurse.
- Treatment without valid consent can led to charges of assault or battery (Pennels, 1997).

Battery

If a patient is touched without their consent, a battery has been committed. A patient's consent may be invalidated if the patient assumes from the nature of the task that the nurse was a doctor. Therefore when carrying out joint injections (a role traditionally performed by doctors), it is important that the patient is clear of the occupational status of the person carrying out the procedure and has consented to this. Unlike negligence, a patient need not exhibit harm to be entitled to bring legal action, but can bring an action if the nurse has behaved in an 'inappropriate' manner causing the patient to experience distress

Table 9.4 Information that the patient requires to make an informed decision

- Details regarding the nature of their condition
- The proposed treatments and alternatives
- The procedure to be undertaken
- Benefits and risks
- Advice regarding after-care

Intra-articular injections

Pharmocokinetics of IA injections

Injectable steroids are synthetic analogues of the adrenal glucocorticoid hormone cortisol, which is secreted by the innermost layer of the adrenal cortex. Corticosteriods influence the production of a wide range of pro-inflammatory mediators, including cytokines, adhesion modules and other enzymes. Although the mechanism of action of injected steroid is not well understood (Owen, 1997), it is primarily used for its anti-inflammatory properties and does have an immunosuppressive component. Corticosteroids facilitate the production of the protein lipocortin, which inhibits the activity of phospholipase A, thus inhibiting the production of inflammatory mediators and reducing inflammation. The steroid is taken up by the synovial cells before being absorbed into the blood and cleared. The synovium is extremely vascular in inflammatory arthritis and the serum concentration of methylprednisolone is related to the number of joints injected rather than the total dose used (Bird, 1998).

Intra-articular corticosteroid preparations

Intra-articular corticosteroids affect the permeability of the synovial membrane (Kay, 1991) – the more insoluble the drug the longer the body takes to remove it, increasing the expected response. Different studies have reported various rates of response following injection of the same agents (Table 9.5).

Blyth et al. (1994) have demonstrated that triamcinolone hexacetonide is the preferred preparation for injection of the knee, with 59% of patients still experiencing improvement in their knee pain at 12 weeks, compared with 44% of patients who received triamcinolone acetonide. Patients who received hydrocortisone in this study required further treatment to their knee. The licensed preparations and routes for injectable corticosteroids are shown in Table 9.6.

Table 9.5 Rates of response to IA corticosteroids

Type of corticosteroid	Response in days
Hydrocortisone acetate	6 (Hollander, 1970) 40 (Rigby et al., 1971)
Triamcinolone hexacetonide	22 (Hollander, 1970) 59 (Rigby et al., 1971) 90 (Anttinen and Oka, 1975)

Table 9.6 Licensed preparations and routes for injectable corticosteroids

Type of corticosteroid	Injectable routes for preparation
Triamcinolone hexacetonide (Lederspan)*	IA, intrasynovial, tendon sheath and bursa, tenosynovitis
Triamcinolone acetonide (Kenalog or Adcortyl)	IA, into bursa, epicondylitis, tenosynovitis
Methylprednisolone acetate (Depo-Medrone)	IA, periarticular, tendon sheath, bursa
Prednisolone acetate (Deltastab)	IA, periarticular, intramuscular, tendon sheath, bursa
Hydrocortisone acetate (Hydrocortistab)	IA, periarticular, intramuscular, tendon sheath, bursa

*Triamcinolone hexacetonide manufacture has been discontinued and it is not currently available in the UK.

The recommended dose range for injectable corticosteroids is shown in Table 9.7

The rationale for administrating IA corticosteroids

Intra-articular corticosteroid can be used for the following purposes:

- Synovitis in a joint (patient should have a recognized inflammatory condition).
- Relief of pain from localized inflammation of a joint.
- Relief of pain in soft tissue disorders, e.g. tennis elbow.
- To supplement systemic disease-modifying anti-rheumatic drug therapy.

Table 9.7 Recommended dose range for injectable corticosteroids

Corticosteroid	Recommended dose (mg)
Dexamethasone (Decadron)	0.4-4 (2-6 for soft tissues)
Triamcinolone hexacetonide (Lederspan) *	2-30
Triamcinolone acetonide (Kenalog or Adcortyl)	Adcortyl 2.5-15
	Kenalog 5-40
Methylprednisolone acetate (Depo-Medrone)	4-80
Prednisolone acetate (Deltastab)	5-25
Hydrocortisone acetate (Hydrocortistab)	5-50 (adults); 5-30 (children)

*Triamcinolone hexacetonide manufacture has been discontinued
and it is not currently available in the UK.

- To improve function/mobilization.
- As a treatment option in patients where the systemic route may be contraindicated, e.g. diabetes or osteoporosis.
- To avoid the need for systemic therapy in patients with monoarthritis, oligoarthritis or isolated soft tissue lesions

With localized disease, consideration should always be given to whether local rest, perhaps enforced by a splint, might remove the need for an injection (Bird, 1998).

The evidence for the use of IA corticosteroid Injections

The literature supports the use of IA corticosteroid injections in the inflammatory arthopathies, where there is subjective and objective improvement in synovitis, as demonstrated by Gray et al. (1981).

The use of IA corticosteroid injections in osteoarthritis (OA) is controversial. Although studies have demonstrated the efficacy of long-acting steroid injections in the knee OA (Dieppe et al., 1980; Gaffney et al., 1995; Jones and Doherty, 1996), there is still doubt about how IA injections should be used for patients with OA. For example, should treatment for pain relief be administered only when there is objective evidence of synovitis? Jones and Doherty (1996) question whether the profession is unduly cautious in the use of IA corticosteroid injections in patients with OA, considering the side effects of non-steroidal anti-inflammatory drugs (NSAIDs) and the lack of evidence indicating cartilage damage (Sparling et al., 1990). Jones and Doherty (1996) propose that all patients with symptomatic OA should be offered a corticosteroid injection to assess response, particularly where anti-inflammatories are contraindicated.

A randomized trial in a primary care population demonstrated that corticosteroid injections administered by GPs for the treatment of a painful, stiff shoulder were superior to physiotherapy (De Wolf and Mens, 1994), due to the quick relief of symptoms occurring in patients treated with an IA injection.

The evidence for local injections in the management of shoulder capsulitis is conflicting. Jacobs et al. (1991) demonstrated that three injections of triamcinolone at 6-weekly intervals was more effective than distension alone in reducing pain and improving passive movements, Whereas Rizk et al. (1991) found that an injection of methylprednisolone and lidocaine (lignocaine) was no more effective than lidocaine alone, except for slight short-lived reduction in pain.

To aspirate or not?

In most rheumatology units, it is routine to aspirate prior to injection and this procedure is well supported by the literature. Aspiration can be useful in the following instances:

- For diagnostic purposes: enabling distinction to be made between inflammatory and non-inflammatory conditions and identifying the presence of infection and crystals. This information, in conjunction with the clinical history and examination, will determine the diagnosis and subsequent treatment.
- In haemoarthrosis or septic arthritis, the blood and infection within the synovial capsule can be toxic and removal is required.
- To ensure correct placement for the injection as well as confirming that frank blood and pus are not present (Dieppe et al., 1980).
- To reduce pain and increase movement (Doherty et al., 1992).
- To reduce the IA pressure, reduce the potentially deleterious effects of the destructive enzymes in the synovial fluid and diminish the dilution factor of the corticosteriod (Neustadt, 1985).
- To improve the benefit of the corticosteroid treatment: Weitoft and Uddenfelt (2000) carried out a prospective study on 147 patients with RA and found that those patients who had received an aspiration prior to the injection of corticosteroid had fewer incidences of arthritis relapse than those patients who had the injection with no aspiration

Table 9.8 describes the constituents of different aspirates.

Some authors (Williams and Gumpel, 1990) advocate leaving synovial fluid in the joint to prevent free diffusion of corticosteroid around the cavity.

Table 9.8 The constituents of aspirated synovial fluid

- Frank blood - often signifies a significant traumatic lesion, e.g. anterior cruciate ligament rupture. It can also occur in the presence of a bleeding disorder or anticoagulant treatment, although this is a relatively rare occurrence
- Fresh blood - a small amount of serous fluid stained with fresh blood is not uncommon and is usually associated with the trauma of aspiration
- Xanthochromic fluid - this is old blood, which appears as an orange colour and signifies an old injury
- Pus - indicates infection, is a rare occurrence and there would be other signs that the patient was unwell
- Straw-coloured fluid - indicates inflammation, commonly seen in patients with RA
- Colourless fluid - indicates normal or non-inflammatory synovial fluid as seen in patients with osteoarthritis
- Milky-white fluid - indicates cholesterol or urate crystals

RA: Rheumatoid Arthritis

Local anaesthetic

In practice, a local anaesthetic is usually administered. It may be pre-injected or mixed with the corticosteroid (Haslock et al., 1995). Experienced clinicians may choose not to use any anaesthetic, as it can be difficult to anaesthetize the capsule and in large joints such as the knee there appears to be no immediate advantage to the patient (Kirwan et al., 1984).

The anaesthetic acts by blocking sodium channels in the nerve to inhibit nerve conduction. The benefits of a local anaesthetic are shown in Table 9.9.

Table 9.9 Potential benefits of local anaesthetic

- Immediate inhibition of inflammatory pain
- Increasing the scope for the effect of the steroid through increasing the volume of the injection, although for small digit joints this may cause painful distension
- Diluting the steroid may reduce the risk of tissue atrophy

There is wide variation between local anaesthetics in terms of their potency, duration of action, toxicity and ability to penetrate the nerve. The effect of lidocaine lasts for approximately one hour, whereas adrenaline lasts for approximately 1.5 hours but is not recommended for use in peripheral joints due to the risk of ischaemia and gangrene. The desirable properties of local anaesthetics are shown in Table 9.10.

Table 9.10 Desirable properties of local anaesthetics

- Non-irritating
- Do not damage the nerve
- Not likely to have systemic effects
- Have a rapid action

Lidocaine is often the drug of choice in IA injections as it has a rapid onset on action (within 5 minutes) and a lower risk of toxicity than adrenaline. It is available in strengths ranging from 0.5% to 2%. Side effects can include:

- facial flushing
- headache and drowsiness
- numbness of the tongue
- blurred vision
- restlessness
- very rare episodes of anaphylaxis/hypotension/bradycardia.

Contraindications to joint injections

Contraindications can be divided into absolute and relative contraindications.

Absolute contraindications

- Trauma or unstable joint.
- Local or systemic infection – an injection in this situation will exacerbate the infection.
- A prosthetic joint, due to the high risk of infection; if indicated it is best performed by a surgeon using full aseptic technique.
- Breakdown in skin integrity.
- Undergoing dental treatment.
- Known allergic reaction.

Relative contraindications

- Diabetes mellitus – corticosteroid can increase blood sugar and the patient will need to know about monitoring their sugar levels closely. If the procedure is required in an unstable diabetic the patient may require hospitalization so that their sugar levels can be monitored.

- Presence of a bleeding disorder or the patient is receiving anticoagulant therapy.
- Doubts regarding the diagnosis.
- Number of previous injections in the site. If numerous injections are being given there is a need to consider overall disease control and alternative interventions.
- Multiple active joint involvement – may be better to use systemic therapy.
- Severe osteoporosis.

Frequency and placement of joint injections

Jones et al. (1993) showed that the placement of IA injections is often inaccurate, especially at the knee and shoulder – the two most commonly injected sites.

There is differing advice in the literature regarding how often injections can be administered and the acceptable time intervals between injections. Cooper and Kirwan (1990) advocate no more than one a month. Swain and Kaplan (1995) have stated a range of 6 to 12 weeks between injections, while Labelle et al. (1992) and Millard and Dillingham (1995) advocate a maximum of three injections per year. It has been argued that providing the interval between injections is not less than four weeks for a weight-bearing joint, the benefit is likely to outweigh the damage by leaving the joint untreated (Balch et al., 1977). A fear of Charcot joints is one of the reasons for restricting the frequency and total number of injections into individual sites, although steroid arthopathy is considered a myth by many clinicians (Cameron, 1995). Evidence linking injected steroids with accelerated nonseptic joint destruction is largely anecdotal. Doherty et al. (1992) state that a reasonable guide is to give injections into weight-bearing joints at no less than three- to four-month intervals, although this advice is based on consensus rather than research evidence. Reports of a Charcot-like destruction in hip osteoarthritis may reflect the disease itself rather than the treatment (Cooper and Kirwan, 1990).

Possible complications of steroid injections

- Joint infection is the most feared side effect and is rare, occurring in 1:50 000 patients (Haslock et al., 1995). Routes of sepsis can include contamination of the injected material, penetration of the skin by organisms, haematogenous spread and reactivation of previous infection. Although staphylococci cause the majority of infections, other organisms including clostridia have also been reported (Seradge and Anderson 1990).

- The most common side effect is facial flushing, occurring in 1:20 patients, which can last for 1-2 days and resolves spontaneously.
- Localized inflammatory flare in the injected joint. This occurrence is supposedly less common with the use of long-acting steroids (Berger and Yoint, 1990). It occurs in about 5% of all injections. Pain can last from one hour to one day. Persistent pain and swelling may indicate missed infection and will require aspiration to identify the infection.
- Diabetic patients can experience a temporary deterioration in diabetic control.
- Subcutaneous atrophy and depigmentation of the skin are more likely to occur when superficial lesions are injected, especially in thin, dark-skinned women (Barry and Jenner, 1995).
- Tendon rupture or atrophy. Current opinion is against injecting steroid into or around the Achilles' tendon (Canoso, 1998). If it is being considered then evidence is required (magnetic resonance imaging (MRI) or ultasound scan) that there is no tear or degenerative changes to the tendon.
- Suppression of the hypothalamic–pituitary–adrenal axis may occur (Reid et al., 1986).
- Irregular menstrual bleeding has been reported (DeWolf and Mens, 1994).
- Patients who are repeatedly injected can be at increased risk of osteoporosis during the injection period. IA steroids are thought to have less effect on bone than oral steroids (Emkey et al., 1996). However, the relative safety of the IA route has not been shown in clinical trials (Canoso, 1998).

Anaphylaxis

For an anaphylactic reaction to occur, the antigen, e.g. corticosteroid and/or lidocaine, must gain entry to the body. Symptoms that may be present in anaphylaxis are shown in Table 9.11. The antigen response that can follow an injection is often more widespread than if the antigen had entered via a different route, i.e. the skin. There can be a generalized vasodilatory effect and increased permeability, with the net effect of loss of intravascular fluid resulting in shock.

Anaphylactic reactions to IA corticosteroid injections

Only 22 cases of allergic reactions following IA or soft tissue corticosteroid injections have been reported in the past 43 years (Mace et al., 1997). These reactions have included hives, hypotension, angio-oedema and bronchospasm. Mace et al. (1997) describe the first case of anaphylaxis

| Table 9.11 Anaphylaxis symptoms | | |

Cutaneous

- swelling (angio-oedema)
- urticaria (hives)
- redness (erythema)
- itching (pruritus)

Central nervous system

- confusion
- feeling of impending doom
- apprehension
- metallic taste
- altered levels of consciousness
- respiratory
- wheezing
- dyspnoea
- rhinitis
- laryngeal obstruction
- hypoxia

Gastrointestinal

- nausea
- diarrhoea
- abdominal cramps
- vomiting

to IA methylprednisolone injection and recommend that, although such events are rare, injectable adrenaline should be kept in the area where this procedure is being performed. Nurses should ensure that they are fully conversant with their local anaphylaxis policy and have had statutory training.

Treatment

No standard treatment algorithm exists for anaphylaxis due to the range of anaphylactic responses that can occur (ILCOR, 1997). In severe cases, the mainstay of treatment is the administration of adrenaline to cause vasoconstriction, thereby increasing the blood pressure and bronchodilatation.

If the patient is exhibiting signs of shock, they will need to be assisted into a prone or semi-recumbent position if airway blockage is suspected. Oxygen should be administered at a high flow rate of 10–15 l/min (ILCOR, 1997) and the patient's vital signs checked. Local hospital practice may include an anaphylaxis policy to enable nurses to administer an injection of adrenaline. Cardiopulmonary resuscitation is sometimes necessary.

The procedure of giving joint injections (Figure 9.1)

Educational preparation

Prior to undertaking soft tissue and joint injections the nurse will require knowledge and skills in the following areas:

- clinical anatomy and physiology
- joint examination
- taking a clinical history
- indications and contraindications for injections
- drug treatments
- patient education
- aspiration and injection techniques
- professional implications of practice.

Figure 9.1 Joint injection. (Silver T (2002) Joint and Soft Tissue Injection (2nd edn). Radcliffe Medical Press, Oxford. Reproduced with permission.)

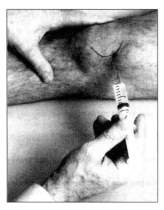
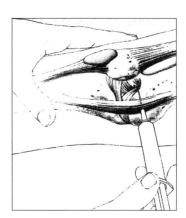

Reproduced with the permission of the copyright holder.

The RCN Rheumatology Forum has guidelines for nurses giving IA injections (see Appendix 4).

Edwards and Hassell (2000) maintain that giving injections without a strong knowledge base in anatomy and physiology and examination techniques demonstrates technical skills only and not true competency in this area of practice.

The aspiration and injection of joints can be performed in an outpatient or inpatient setting and should incorporate a number of stages (Table 9.12).

Table 9.12 Procedural steps in IA administration

- The procedure must be explained to the patient and informed consent obtained
- The patient should be placed in a comfortable position; this is usually on a couch
- Hands must be washed thoroughly
- An aseptic/non-touch technique is used to protect the patient. The importance of a non-touch technique is recognized by the majority of clinicians, although there is a lack of consensus as to what the term means (Haslock et al., 1995)
- Gloves should be worn to protect the practitioner, although this was an uncommon practice by the rheumatologists surveyed by Haslock et al. (1995)
- The area for the injection is inspected and palpated. Some practitioners use a thumbnail cross to identify the entry site
- The steroid and anaesthetic for administration are drawn up; the name of the preparation, dose and expiry date are checked
- The needle is changed after drawing up the drug
- The skin is cleaned thoroughly with an antiseptic agent. There is no consensus concerning skin preparation techniques prior to IA injection (Cawley and Morris, 1992). A postal survey of consultant rheumatologists confirmed widespread differences in clinical practice (Haslock et al., 1995). Cawley and Morris (1992) demonstrated that there was no bacteriological superiority of chlorhexidine in spirit over isopropyl alcohol swipe; however, the use of an alcohol swipe had an economic advantage
- With the proper technique the needle passes through the extra-articular tissues and a 'pop' is felt as the needle enters the joint. Accurate needle placement is important for clinical efficacy and to avoid adverse reactions (Jones et al., 1993)
- It is important to establish if aspirate is present; if it is, it is removed. Several factors can influence the aspiration. If the aspiration is proving difficult it may be necessary to rotate the needle or withdraw the syringe slightly (see Figure 9.1 and Table 9.13). Once the aspirate is removed the injection can be administered through the same needle but via a different syringe
- Never inject if resistance is present (in IA injections resistance usually indicates that the needle is in a tendon)
- At the end of the procedure the needle should be withdrawn and a plaster applied for a few hours
- Ensure safe disposal of sharps

Table 9.13 Factors influencing the aspiration (Canoso, 1998)

- Size of the needle
- Viscosity of the fluid
- Amount of synovitis
- Presence of fibrin clots

Documentation

Many nurses are giving IA injections under the guidance of patient group directions, which will be replaced by supplementary prescribing in 2003 (DoH, 2003a). It is important that the following information is recorded in the patient documentation:

- Assessment and rationale for injecting joint.
- How consent was obtained.
- The site injected, along with the name and dosage of the preparation and the approach used (e.g. medial).
- Whether any aspirate was obtained and, if so, the amount and appearance and whether it was sent for culture.
- Post-injection advice and follow-up care – this may be given in the form of an information leaflet.

After-care

There is a great deal of variation in the advice given (Canoso, 1998). Patients need to be provided with both verbal and written information. The Arthritis and Rheumatism Campaign (arc) produces a leaflet entitled 'Drugs for arthritis – local steroid injections' (see Appendix 5). If you are developing your own leaflet, the following aspects, as suggested by Hill (1998), need to be considered:

- Use lay terminology. It is a good idea to check local trust policy on developing information sheets, which might include the involvement of a patient panel in the development of all patient information.
- Write in short paragraphs.
- Use one- or two-syllable words if possible.
- Adopt a question-and-answer format.
- Use positive language
- Refer to trust policies and guidelines where appropriate.

The joint may be painful for 24–48 hours, so the patient should be advised to use analgesia as required, and to contact the department if they experience fever, joint swelling or joint redness. The additional use of splinting may be advocated following injection in soft tissue conditions of the hand and wrist.

Intra-articular injections can cause a significant fall in the erythrocyte sedimentation rate (ESR) and C-reactive protein (CRP) levels. This needs to be taken into account when using blood tests to assess the efficacy of DMARDs or biologic therapies.

Rest

The literature advocates rest (Cooper and Kirwan, 1990) relative to the site of the injection. There is consensus that it is sensible for the patient to rest the weight-bearing joints for 24–48 hours to minimize leakage of the agent and to improve the anti-inflammatory response. Some clinicians arrange admission for bed rest (Haslock et al., 1995). There are no studies indicating whether bed rest prevents Charcot joints, although there is some evidence that it increases the efficacy of the procedure (Chakravarty et al., 1994). It is thought that partial immobilization of the injected joint inhibits the absorptive capacity of the synovial membrane and delays systemic effects (Jones et al., 1993). Patients are also advised to restrict activities that can cause symptoms, although no particular time frame is given (Jacobs et al., 1991; Neustadt, 1991). Following a shoulder injection the advice would be to restrain from shoulder activities, e.g. racquet sports, for 10–14 days.

Why might an IA injection fail to relieve the symptoms for which it is administered?

- Poor technique – the injection was given in the wrong place.
- Incorrect diagnosis made.
- Difficult area to inject – may need to use x-ray control to ensure that the injection is in the right place.
- Not all patients experience symptomatic benefit.

Audit of nurse-led practice

The first joint injection course for nurses approved by the English National Board was established at Cannock Chase Hospital in 1995, and over 50 nurses have now completed this course (Edwards et al., 2002). In 1999, the course leaders sent out questionnaires to all course participants (n = 36; 21 responded) to assess the impact of the course on nursing practice. All the respondents claimed still to be injecting joints, with 15 nurses injecting more than four times each month (Edwards and Hassell, 2000).

Edwards et al. (2002) performed an audit of all patients who underwent an IA or soft tissue injection in one rheumatology department over a month. A total of 170 corticosteroid injections were given to 103 patients. Nurses gave 114 (67%) of these injections to 63 patients. Sites injected by the nurses included ankle, wrist, knee, elbow, glenohumeral and sub-acromial injections. The medical staff gave all subtalar and carpometacarpal joint injections. Overall satisfaction of injections given by nurses and doctors was similar, with a mean visual analogue score (VAS) of 8 for the nurses (range 1.1–10) and 7.8 for the doctors (range 0.6–10). This level of satisfaction demonstrated by the patient for nurse adminis-tration of IA injections is replicated in many in-house (unpublished) audits in other rheumatology departments. Joint injections are undertaken by other health professionals with extended roles, including physiotherapists and podiatrists. A CD-ROM exploring clinical anatomy and examination using an interactive learning format is available from the Arthritis and Rheumatism Campaign (arc).

Conclusions

Chronic disease nursing is an area where the nurse will need to utilize both instrumental and expressive skills to benefit patient care. Prior to undertaking any new role component, the nurse must be aware of the legal and professional requirements of role extension. The profession should endorse new role development that improves patient care.

Table of cases

Bolam v Friern Hospital Management Committee (1957) 1 WLR 582

Chapter 10

Leadership and clinical governance

Jill Bryne and Georgina Clark

Introduction

As leaders of clinical services we need to have assurances, through a clinical governance system, that the care we provide is of the highest quality, evidence based and patient centred (DoH, 2002a). Clinical governance cannot be effective in the absence of leaders and champions, who will continually promote its importance on a day-to-day basis.

It is for this reason that this chapter has two sections. The first provides an overview of the leadership skills that will be needed to develop and sustain service improvement, and the second offers practical guidance about the implementation of a clinical governance framework.

Figure 10.1 illustrates how quality services are supported by the pillars of clinical governance. In turn, this is underpinned by strong leadership from staff who have a vision for the future of healthcare.

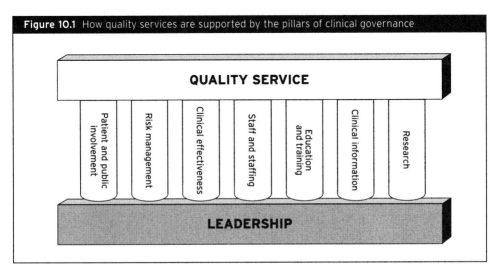

Figure 10.1 How quality services are supported by the pillars of clinical governance

QUALITY SERVICE

Patient and public involvement

Risk management

Clinical effectiveness

Staff and staffing

Education and training

Clinical information

Research

LEADERSHIP

This chapter provides:

- an overview of essential aspects of leadership needed to recognize and support a clinical governance framework
- examples of tools to support nurses developing leadership skills
- an overview of clinical governance and guidance on implementing quality improvements
- practical information on the seven pillars of clinical governance
- examples to demonstrate quality improvements using the seven pillars of clinical governance.

Leadership and clinical governance

The aim of this section is to provide an overview of some tools and techniques that an effective leader can use to assist them in leading the development of a new service. Clinical governance can be effective only if championed by strong leadership. The areas examined are:

- leadership
- role development
- communication
  - business planning
  - chairing meetings
- change management
- dealing with people
- multidisciplinary working
- conflict management
- environmental profiling.

Leadership

Background

The NHS is an ever-changing environment, and there is a need for people with specific attributes to take the lead in this environment. However, not all excellent clinicians are born leaders and hence they need support in developing effective leadership skills when in a more strategic leadership role.

There are a number of identified and documented leadership qualities and often they are phrased in different ways or have a different emphasis, depending on the organizational needs or theoretical models discussed. Some examples of leadership qualities include creativity, self-awareness and enthusiasm (Tremblay and Dunn, 2002). Three areas that are often highlighted in leadership theory are those of:

- strategy, developing a sense of purpose and direction for the staff
- defining what is necessary for the team to achieve their goals effectively
- interpersonal skills needed to motivate the team, and maintain morale and commitment of the group (Adair, 1982) (Figure 10.2).

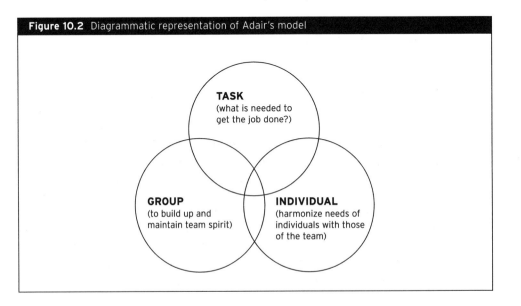

Figure 10.2 Diagrammatic representation of Adair's model

Practical steps

- **Mentorship**: using a role model is a good way of developing leadership skills. Find someone who you respect either inside or outside the organization and ask if they would act as a mentor.
- **Professional development for the leader**: it has been recognized nationally that effective leadership is vital to lead nursing into this century. Hence many resources have been invested into developing leaders. These include the Royal College of Nursing (RCN) Leadership Programme, Leading Empowered Organizations (LEO) programmes run by the National Nursing Leadership Programme (NNLP) and the Modernisation Agency (DoH, 2002a). A nursing leadership website has been developed that provides a broad range of tools that offer personal development, theoretical models and a step-wise approach to managing as a leader (www.nursing-leadership.co.uk).

- **Shadowing**: some of the most effective learning experiences lie outside the formal education arena. These can be a cost-effective way of professional development. As with mentorship, it is important to find people with roles that provide a learning opportunity. Time spent working alongside them during daily clinical practice often provides valuable experiences that are difficult to achieve in a classroom setting. If it works well then the experience can be cascaded to others in the team, acting as a catalyst for their development.

Role development of the team

Background

When establishing a new team, it important to recognize the value of the staff working within that service. Roles within the team need to be clearly identified, as failure to do so can have a devastating effect on job performance, leading to poor staff retention and increased absenteeism. Failure to clarify roles and responsibilities can lead to poor motivation and lack of commitment to the organization's aims and objectives.

It is recognized nationally that there is a need to promote an increased contribution from nursing within the NHS, but this needs to be developed within a safe and consistent framework (DoH, 1999a). Technological developments in rheumatology have inevitably resulted in nurses performing more advanced and specialist roles. As a service leader, you will need to consider a balance between developing practice and the safety of both patients and staff.

In order to develop roles, team members may be keen to impress and may take on new tasks and skills. However, this willingness must be balanced against accountability and vicarious liability. Similarly, it is unfair and inappropriate for an organization to expect or allow a nurse to practise beyond her competency, outside of protocols and/or without the appropriate training

Practical steps

- Understand exactly what the service wants to achieve and discuss/document this.
- How will the development of the role enhance the service?
- Identify how the patients/users will benefit from this role.
- Get an idea of what is done elsewhere (visit other units).
- Ensure that protocols and policies are developed.
- Develop a comprehensive job description, from specification and job plan.

- Develop the service in a step-by-step process at a pace that the team can manage..
- Establish a system of role review.
- Ensure support and development opportunities are available to the person in this role.
- Consider professional guidance. For example, *The NHS Plan* identified the need for breaking down barriers between professionals, leading to the modernization of the nursing role (DoH, 2000a). The Chief Nursing Officer's ten key roles for nurses set out in *The NHS Plan* can be seen in Appendix 1.

Communication

Effective communication is key to the implementation of clinical governance. In most circumstances, nurses demonstrate exceptional communication skills with patients. However, nurses can be subjective in their approach to describing patient experience and service needs. Specific skills need to be considered when establishing new services. This section includes several areas, for example business planning and chairing meetings.

Business planning/report writing

When compiling a case for service development the contribution must be as objective as possible and evidence-based. Each organization will have its own preferred method of business planning; the best way to find out the format is to contact your line manager or corporate planning department. The main facets of a business care or report are described in Chapter 2.

Meetings

As a leader, responsibilities will often include attending meetings and regular communication with others. Valuable time and vital information can be lost if meetings are poorly chaired. Chairing meetings can be a terrifying experience but using some simple pointers the process can be made easier (see Challinor, 1999).

Practical steps
- Preparation is the key to good meetings, so care and attention should be paid to the purpose of the meeting, who is attending, the frequency and length of the meeting.

- When attending a meeting, ensure that you read information in advance. Prepare thoroughly, with relevant facts readily available to refer to. At the meeting, ensure that you note down key facts discussed to aid recall of the important points while waiting for minutes of the meeting to be typed. Also, use your expertise and skill appropriately by choosing the most opportune time to make a statement or contribute information to the group. Be succinct.
- Meetings can be monopolized by a small number of people with strong personalities, or alternatively can focus on trivialities rather than the issues in hand. To ensure effective outcomes the chair needs to maintain direction, have an organized structure to the meeting and ensure clarity of decision making. Table 10.1 identifies the key points to consider when chairing meetings so that they run smoothly.

Table 10.1 Considerations for meetings

- Define the objectives of the meeting
- Set a timescale
- Develop an agenda and circulate it prior to the meeting
- At the meeting, go through each item on the agenda
- Ensure that a firm conclusion/action is reached and recorded
- Initiate discussions ensuring that all parties are involved
- Encourage expression of different views

Change management

Change is a constant process, which exists everywhere and happens in all aspects of our lives. Some changes are quick (these can be called operational) and others are longer term (strategic).

People react differently to change; some accept it well while others find change very difficult. It is important when making changes to consider the impact that the changes will have on anyone involved.

Practical steps

- Iles and Sutherland (2001) use a 'project management' model for managing change. The phases of this model can be seen in Table 10.2.

Dealing with people

Background

Hospitals employ a cross-section of staff with varying personal and professional priorities as well as differing professional backgrounds. In some

Table 10.2 Phases of project management

Areas to identify	Action required
Purpose	Why is the change needed?
Definition	An outline of what the change seeks to achieve
Plan	Develop a plan or map identifying the specific steps needed and associated timescales; include activities and resources that are needed to achieve this plan
Monitoring	Ensure that progress is regularly assessed. Review the long-term objectives and progress; if problems are identified develop corrective plans
Evaluation	On completion of the project (change), an evaluation of the change and objectives achieved should be undertaken

Adapted from Iles and Sutherland (2001).

multidisciplinary teams, the nurse specialist may not have line management responsibility for the staff yet is expected to assist the group in achieving unified team working. Without this control, collaboration is needed to strengthen partnership and motivate the team to meet objectives (Parker, 1990).

Multidisciplinary team working

It is useful to assess the varying levels of power and influence within the team and find ways of securing everyone's support. This is called 'stakeholder analysis', and is described in more detail by Iles and Sutherland (2001), who use this method to identify the driving forces and limiting forces that relate to change.

It is also useful to understand the theoretical models of team dynamics, as the stages of team performance are constantly changing. Team dynamics and performance have been described in five stages:

- Forming - individuals are cautious, looking for a leader and direction.
- Storming - frustration and anger as deadlines loom and perspectives clash.

- Norming – become more sensitive to other members of team.
- Performing – oriented to task and team, pulling together, good communication.
- Adjourning – review of completed work, set action plans.

For more information go to www.nursingleadership.co.uk

A model of power highlights three influences on positive power (Claus and Bailey, 1997). These are:

- strength – awareness of one's own ability and skills
- energy – the will to respond and act, and positively
- action – 'powerful' person acts in order to solve problems or make a decision.

Whenever groups of people work together towards an identified goal, the influence of power and control within the team cannot be ignored. However much it is resisted, becoming involved in the politics of a situation, and power and politics are everyday aspects of our work. There is a need to be knowledgeable about the potential impact on service provision.

Table 10.3 Dealing with conflict

Phase	Action
1 Peaceful coexistence	This is when the individuals learn to live with each other and are helped to smooth out some difficulties and identify common ground
2 Compromise	In this situation neither party wins or loses and a compromise is achieved by negotiation
3 Problem solving	In this approach an attempt is made to find a genuine solution rather than to accommodate different views

Adapted from Armstrong (1994).

Conflict management

It is inevitable that from time to time there will be conflict, and this conflict can be essential for change and progress to occur. Conflict can present from a line manager, colleague or supporting staff, and can arise for various reasons, ranging from a misunderstanding or a difference in values and beliefs to a clash of personalities. Sometimes it can occur simply because feelings and emotions are running high.

Whatever the cause, it has been suggested that there are three ways to deal with conflict (Armstrong, 1994) (Table 10.3).

Environmental assessment

Background

Nurses use models of care to make an assessment of a patient's condition on a daily basis. The aim of assessment models is to ensure that all relevant factors are given equal weighting and are objective. The principles are no different when leading a service – it is simply the assessment tool that changes. As with nursing models, the tools available to influence organizations vary. Some tools have been specifically designed with business planning processes in mind.

The team leader needs to think clearly and continually to sift through the information, selecting what is relevant and examining how these factors interact. Using specific management 'tools' (e.g. the five stages of team performance) can help to clarify the potential priorities and pressures within the multidisciplinary team as well as within the service organization and beyond. Two models are outlined in this chapter:

- the social, technological, economic, environmental, political (STEEP) model (Brocklehurst et al., 1999)
- a strengths, weaknesses, opportunities and threats (SWOT) analysis.

STEEP model

This is an environmental research tool historically used in marketing, whch is used to scan, monitor, forecast and assess the environment, taking five factors into consideration, as shown in Table 10.4. There are variations of this model with different acronyms, but the theme remains the same – that of evaluating the environmental issues that affect development.

SWOT analysis

SWOT analysis is a tool developed in the 1960s for examining an organization's strengths, weaknesses, opportunities and threats and thus aid identification of priorities for action (Iles and Sutherland, 2001). A model of this can be seen in Figure 10.3. Iles and Sutherland (2001) identify questions to ask when considering strengths and weaknesses, and the opportunities and threats, and are incorporated in Figure 10.3.

Table 10.4 STEEP model

Factors	Questions to ask
Social	• What is happening in the local community? • Is there an aged population? • What do the public think of the service?
Technological	• What technological/pharmacological interventions are occurring that will change practice? • Is there any recent audit and research that impacts on your service? • Are there any new ways of working that will influence practice (i.e. NICE guidelines, College of Rheumatology guidelines)?
Economic	• What budgeting factors need to be considered? • Is your service cost-effective? • Are there sufficient monies in the system to purchase new and expensive drugs?
Environmental	• What environmental factors need to be considered (i.e. changes within PCTs, trust mergers, SHAs)?
Political	• How might politics influence the rheumatology service? • Who are the 'key players' and where is the power base?

Figure 10.3 SWOT analysis

Positive factors	Negative factors	
Strengths	Weaknesses	Internal factors
• What are the consequences of this? • Do they help or hinder in achieving the aim?		
Opportunities	Threats	External factors
• What impact is this likely to have on us? • Will it help or hinder?		

Conclusions

It is important to recognize that not everyone wants, or has the ability, to take on leadership roles. However, sometimes certain leadership attributes may need to be developed or learnt in order to effect the change or development that is hoped for. It is important to have knowledge of leadership styles and models applied in management. It will enable aspiring leaders to identify personal attributes or weaknesses that may need refinement or inform reflection on aspects of current leadership style and whether they have been successful. Equally they will inform those who do not wish to lead but recognize the elements that lead to success in management and the individuals' responsibility in supporting leaders. As individuals, it is possible to develop personal expertise or find ways of supporting or guiding others in this challenging role.

To have a motivated team that works in a safe and effective manner, good leadership is essential. The culture of good leadership is one that should be applied at an individual and organizational level and it is a key component for the successful implementation of effective clinical governance frameworks, as described below.

Clinical governance

Clinical governance has been described as:

> A framework through which NHS organisations are accountable for continually improving the quality of their services and safeguard high standards of care by creating an environment in which excellence in clinical care will flourish (Scally and Donaldson, 1998).

Clinical governance is a framework that sets out to identify a whole-system approach to the delivery of high-quality care. Healthcare professionals working within this framework use evidence-based care, working at a high standard, reducing risks and hazards, and creating a safe and effective culture. This means that patient-centred care should be at the forefront of decision making, ensuring accurate information and documentation with processes and outcomes that are accessible to all.

Patient and public involvement

Background

Patient and public involvement (PPI) describes a process by which patients, carers and the public are actively encouraged to voice their opinions about

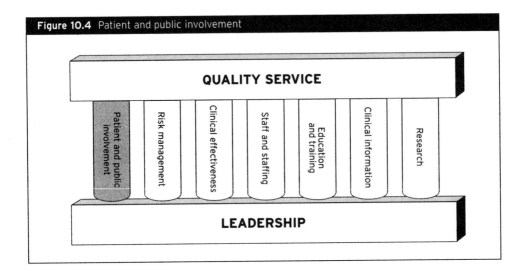

Figure 10.4 Patient and public involvement

their experiences of healthcare. Used effectively this process can direct service development and modernization, e.g. design of ward layouts, clinic times, hospital menus. If the feedback is negative, an openness to criticism teamed with a willingness to listen will result in some excellent changes to practice, some of which are discussed later in this section

Among the key factors that have driven PPI were the recommendations that led from the Bristol Royal Inquiry, which recommended that there should be representation of patients' interests 'on the inside' of the NHS at every level. It must also be remembered that, as a public service, NHS user customers have the right to know that they are receiving quality care that is safe, clinically effective and value for money.

In response to this a new system has been established for PPI in England (Health and Social Care Act 2001: DoH, 2001f; NHS Reform and Healthcare Professions Act 2002: DoH, 2002c). The new national structure will result in the following changes:

- Community Health Councils (CHCs) will be abolished as of September 2003.
- Patient Advice and Liaison Service (PALS) and patient forums will be set up in every NHS trust and primary care trust (PCT), to influence the day-to-day management of health services.
- A new Commission for Patient and Public Involvement in Health (CPPIH) will establish, support and facilitate the co-ordination of the patient forums.
- Patients can be involved, if they wish to be, in decisions about their services and health.

Although nurses recognize the importance of listening to patients, formal mechanisms to ensure this happens and that information gained is acted upon are often lacking. Services must demonstrate that they put the patient at the centre of everything they do, and frameworks need to be in place to support this.

Consideration must also be given to involving the patient with regard to:

- obtaining consent
- resuscitation.

These two issues require the highest standards of patient consultation and are probably two of the biggest 'minefield' areas for nurses, allied health professionals and doctors. The new guidelines on consent that were issued were accompanied by a new format of consent form and protocol for obtaining consent (DoH, 2001e). Table 10.6 poses questions to help teams reflect on consent issues.

Table 10.6 Team approach

Questions

- Are team members familiar with the new consent guidance?
- Are the new consent forms in use in the clinic or wards?
- Is the consenting professional, e.g. nurse, allied healthcare professional or doctor appropriately trained?
- Does the patient have enough information to give 'informed' consent?
- Has the patient been provided with the most updated evidenced-based patient information for him or her to gain this knowledge?

Practical steps

Gather support from others.

- Link with your PALS department for advice. Despite being new departments they are developing a wealth of information on PPI. Ask them to come and talk to the team/department. Their examples of changes that have been made as a result of comments made can be very inspiring.
- If the trust has a strategy for PPI, read it, it might offer you ideas and avoid reinvention of the wheel. It may be appropriate to write a 'vision paper' or strategy for rheumatology on how the service involves users.
- Contact the CPPIH for additional support on how to set up user groups.

Developing structures to promote PPI

- Consider establishing a patient forum/opinion group. Brainstorm with the clinical team to find out what agenda they think the patients would find useful.
- Introduce a PPI notice board in the clinic with suggestion cards and a box for posting, using the supermarket concept of 'You Told Us and We Changed'.
- Some departments have developed monthly inpatient forums. All patients were invited to join the nurses in the ward lounge and, over coffee, were asked to share their experiences of their inpatient stay. The concept is simple and low maintenance but the feedback can be enlightening!

PPI is an ideal tool to promote multidisciplinary working and involvement of non-qualified staff. Health support workers have initiated and managed some excellent examples of patient involvement. The feedback is rich and can be challenging, but there is also likely to be very positive feedback for staff. There is a wealth of examples that can be used to highlight the success of PPI. Some are sophisticated, others are on a much simpler scale, as can be seen in the following example:

- A pharmacy display has been introduced in the outpatient waiting area in one hospital to describe the dispensing process for outpatients, following complaints reflecting unclear patient expectations.

Pillar: risk management

Background

Rheumatology services in the modern NHS see more patients, often with a shorter length of stay and more complex therapies provided by nurses and doctors working in more advanced roles. Under these circumstances it is easy to envisage that there is a greater potential for clinical error. All errors have potentially massive implications:

- The personal cost to the patient of clinical injury.
- The cost to the organization – in terms of litigation.

All healthcare professionals have a responsibility to ensure that the patient's journey through the healthcare system is managed with the least possible risk. This has to be achieved by vigilance in the assessment of risk and proactive management to ensure that risks (or potential risks) are removed or reduced to acceptable levels for the patient and the organization.

Historically staff have been fearful of admitting to mistakes and there is a need to promote an open culture, encouraging health professionals to

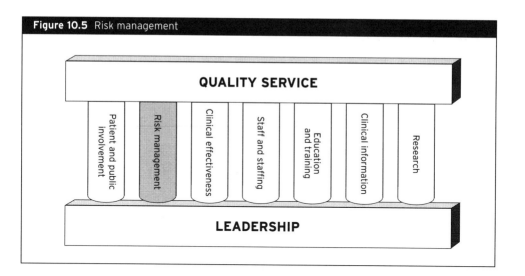

Figure 10.5 Risk management

report incidents and 'near misses'. Staff should be encouraged to report incidents without fear of personal reprimand and know that others will be able to learn from their experiences and improve patient safety.

The organization's risk team will collate incidents from clinical areas, using the results to highlight areas where trends show increased risk. From an organizational point of view this can be used to allocate additional resources or support and inform the business planning process for the hospital, ensuring that the areas of greater risk are given the highest priority.

There are three key areas to consider.

- Incident reporting – the best organizations have the highest incident reporting rate, reported by staff who feel comfortable to do so.
- Risk assessment – there is a need to know where specific risks lie and to prioritize them by allocating a score and acting to remedy or accept the risk.
- Consider how the service can learn from mistakes and near misses.

The National Patient Safety Agency (NPSA) was established to collate incidents into a national database and facilitate NHS-wide learning from incidents (NPSA, 2002).

Practical steps

- Read the trust's risk management strategy.
- Ensure that all staff have risk management training.

Table 10.7 Risk management

Questions

- Who is responsible for co-ordinating clinical risk in the department, directorate or trust?
- What training is available to staff to support risk management?
- Has the service been risk assessed?
- What systems are in place for reporting clinical incidents and near misses?
- What changes have occurred as a result of incidents?

- Ask the clinical risk department to talk to the team. They can offer support on carrying out risk assessments, and how to scrutinize all the various procedures and activities carried out in the area, and identify the possible risks and grade them according to their potential frequency and severity.
- Share the evidence of any changes to practice that might have resulted from reported clinical incidents and 'near misses'.

An example of a change to practice by a trust:

- A series of incidents and complaints about a clinical team's attitude to patients has resulted in the development by the trust of a specific customer care training programme.

Pillar: staff and staff training

Background

A successful service will be dependent on a motivated and dedicated team who will strive to provide the highest standards of patient-centred care.

For staff to achieve their full potential, they need to feel nurtured, respected and involved in all aspects of the service provision. In addition, all members of the team need to feel confident in their capabilities and competencies. Training can in part provide this, although it is likely that the leader of the team will provide the most powerful impact when working as a role model to others. Success will also be dependent on how the nurse (or leader) develops, appraises and supports the team.

Practical steps

- Communication – it is vital that large organizations have effective channels of communication. Nurse managers will need to be confident that all the team receive the essential information to enable them to provide safe standards of care. This starts with the production of clear local policies, regularly updated in accordance with current evidence-based practice.

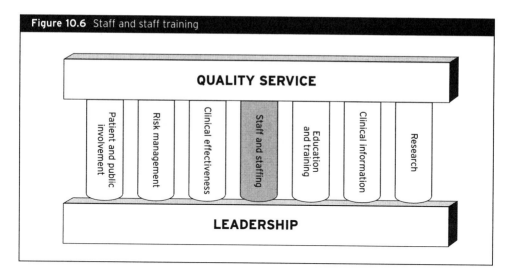

Figure 10.6 Staff and staff training

QUALITY SERVICE

Patient and public involvement

Risk management

Clinical effectiveness

Staff and staffing

Education and training

Clinical information

Research

LEADERSHIP

There should also be effective communication routes all the way, from the executive team to every member of staff. The manager/leader is the vital link who co-ordinates both 'top-down' and 'bottom-up' communication. In addition, once key workers are in receipt of information, it is essential that they disseminate to the team in an interesting and effective manner.

- Staff induction – all new staff must have participated in local and corporate induction so that they have an awareness of how the department and organization function.
- Appraisal – effective managers will recognize the need for all staff (including the manager) to be regularly appraised. This provides an opportunity to consider the following questions:
  - What is my job?
  - How am I doing?
  - What do I need to develop?

Table 10.8 Staff and staff development

Questions

- What are the arrangements for induction, including temporary staff?
- Are there regular appraisals for staff?
- Is there a system for ensuring that staff are appropriately qualified and have the opportunity for clinical supervision?
- What can be expected from the team and how will poor performance be dealt with if they fall short of these expectations?
- Have appropriate numbers and skill-mix of staff for the service been identified?

Clinical governance reviews conducted by the Commission for Health Improvement (CHI) have highlighted that many staff are not appraised and standards of appraisals vary across trusts. If uncertain of any aspect of the process, check with the human resources/personnel department, trust websites or policy folder where most of the guidance for appraisal might be found.

- Clinical supervision – the value of the individual within an organization can be demonstrated by the commitment to clinical supervision. Supervision can be extremely effective in enabling staff to reach their full potential and can take the form of one-to-one interviews or group sessions. There is a plethora of information to support and establish various frameworks for supervision (Brocklehurst and Walsh, 1999).
- Dealing with poor performance – professionals have a responsibility to report and/or deal with poor performance. It is one of the most difficult tasks that faces any professional, and expert support should be sought if needed. Ideally, issues should be addressed locally and as soon as they arise through the trust's performance management framework. Regulatory bodies such as the Nursing and Midwifery Council (NMC) can provide specific guidance and support.
- Staffing levels and skill-mix – staffing levels and skill-mix are the determining factors in the level and standard of service that can be provided. Unfortunately there is little national guidance on how to determine appropriate staffing levels for a service. Within a given budget it is imperative that the appropriate skill-mix is secured if the care provided is to be of a desired standard.

Pillar: education and training

Background

Developing a new service needs more than enthusiasm and vision. A team is required that is prepared to show its initiative and 'go the extra mile'. The service is only as strong as the team and therefore it is wise to invest in the training of the team.

Nurses will need to be confident that the team has the appropriate skills to carry out the role that it has been appointed to do. The organisation should recognize the value of investing in the team to ensure that they are committed and confident that they have the appropriate skills to achieve identified goals.

How will the required skills be identified? The clinical core competencies and knowledge base needed for rheumatology nurses is reasonably well documented, but the individual's level of expertise needs to be accurately assessed.

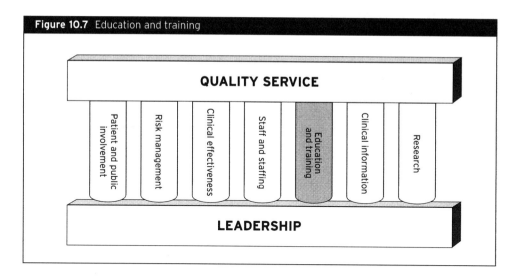

Figure 10.7 Education and training

By identifying individual training needs through appraisal, hospitals can build a training programme that ensures that staff can achieve their objectives. This also needs to be done at a local level. Effective organization of appraisal enables a focused approach to examining the team needs and planning appropriate training.

Other factors that may influence planning needs and provide a clear direction for training needs or review of areas of high risk include:

- feedback from patients
- clinical incident reporting
- complaints, results of coroner's inquests and clinical negligence claims.

There are statutory training needs essential to all staff irrespective of grade, and these will form the mandatory or compulsory programme, e.g. moving and handling, fire safety. The employer has a responsibility to provide these for all employees.

There will also be special skills required for specific groups, for example rheumatology nurses. Specialist training can be extortionately expensive and the value of the courses in both purpose and cost-effectiveness needs to be considered.

Practical steps

- **Formal courses or study days** are not always the most effective routes of education. Look for non-formal methods of education.
- **Consider arranging 'shadowing' experiences** for all members of the team. Insights gained from sharing clinical experiences can broaden

---

Table 10.9 Education and training

Questions

- Are appropriate nursing staff experienced in appraisal techniques and have they established an appraisal programme?
- Is there a programme for work-based training, i.e. developing professional portfolio?
- Who is responsible for and what support is there for staff training (funds, protected time, libraries) and is there an established appraisal programme?
- Is there a training programme or prospectus for staff training?
- What systems are there to ensure that mandatory training requirements are met?

---

experience and develop teamworking. Equally, a team member can shadow an identified lead attending meetings or visiting units/organizations. It offers a perfect opportunity for others to see the role at closer proximity. It also provides a dedicated one-to-one session following the 'shadowing' to answer more specific issues.

- **Ensure prompt appraisal** of the new team. The review process may identify several members of the team who have similar training needs. It is far more cost- and time-effective to provide education in a group than to meet individual needs separately. So, for example, if there is a need to understand more about a new drug therapy, ask the pharmacy department to consider some in-house training. This will not only be 'free', but will be specific to the needs of the team.
- **Value for money** – ensure that courses are evaluated effectively and not reliant on anecdotal evidence. Review the course from a quality as well as a cost-effectiveness perspective, ideally through past candidates. Before looking outside the organization check in-house courses. Courses require a commitment from specific work areas (or units) as well as the employing organization. This will require recognition that the individual will be released to attend courses as well as possible funding issues in providing temporary replacement staff. Equally, the individual attending a course has a responsibility to cascade their newly acquired knowledge or skill.
- **Network with other units** – link with other hospitals and colleagues to see what training they have found effective. Explore training opportunities through professional and specialist groups. Consider establishing a local network for training.
- **Mandatory training** programmes are compiled from those areas of healthcare that pose the greatest risk to patients and staff alike. For example, if members of the team consistently fail to attend fire lectures, the potential impact for the hospital and patients is significant. Staff must attend and the lead for the service has professional responsibility to ensure that this happens.

- **Understanding the wider picture** – anecdotally, it is felt that the majority of the clinical workforce is not aware of the clinical governance agendas and do not understand the trust objectives. An example is that of key performance indicators against which hospitals are performance managed. Many have never read the NHS National Plan (DoH, 2000a) or the national nursing strategy *Making a Difference* (DoH, 1999a). In truth, many clinicians tend to catch up with the wider picture of healthcare when required to, e.g. when preparing for interviews, etc. Look for opportunities to involve staff in the political and wider healthcare agenda. To practise in isolation of the wider context will not enable staff to be informed or become effective ambassadors for the service.

An example of a practical step:

- One trust noted that there was an increased incident of complaints from patients/relatives about how bad news was given to them by doctors. In response, they developed a 'Breaking Bad News' training programme.

Use of clinical information – the value to clinical care

Background

Information is very powerful and can be used to assist decision making and business planning. It informs thought processes to ensure that objective decisions are made. Nurses are sometimes criticized for being subjective and reacting from the heart. Good, accurate information will provide the evidence to support a case when striving to develop patient services.

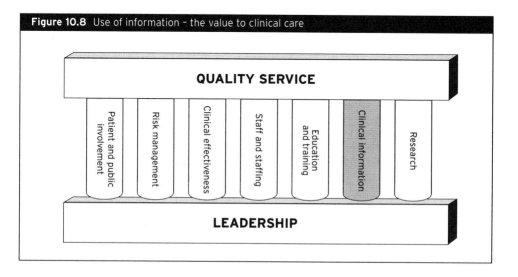

Figure 10.8 Use of information – the value to clinical care

QUALITY SERVICE

Patient and public involvement | Risk management | Clinical effectiveness | Staff and staffing | Education and training | Clinical information | Research

LEADERSHIP

Information comes in many formats and skill is needed to access, analyse and utilize this information to its full potential. Clinical information is collected at many levels. Individual organizations within the NHS are performance managed against a series of key performance indicators. Trusts have a responsibility to collect specific data for the strategic health authority (SHA) to guide performance reviews of the NHS. This information is analysed and trusts are star rated according to their success in achieving these performance targets. Accurate information is therefore essential.

Many clinical services are not aware of the data that are collected about them. For example, the trust's information department will have figures on:

- the number of patients attending the service
- the length of time that they wait for appointments
- the length of stay for inpatients
- the cost of admissions/treatment per patient
- the number of procedures performed.

In addition, vital data are collected from clinical audit, benchmarking research, patients' complaints, satisfaction surveys and comments to PALS, which are all key to decision making within the service.

Table 10.10 Clinical information

Questions

- Has the hospital/trust had a review from the Commission for Health Improvement (CHI)? If so, read the report; it will provide an oversight into their progress with clinical governance (www.chi.gov.uk)
- What information is there about patients' experiences of care (e.g. complaint, satisfaction surveys)?
- How is information accessed about the performance of the service within the organization?
- How are professionals informed on achievements of objectives, i.e. how is information used to demonstrate performance?
- What changes to practice have occurred as a result of this information?
- What systems are in place to ensure confidentiality of information?

Practical steps

- The NHS Information Authority (NHSIA) has a wealth of information available to support practitioners on clinical governance issues. A user-friendly website identifies a broad range of information which can inform or support healthcare professionals (see Appendix 2).

- Identify information collected about the specific service area of interest (e.g. respiratory). There will be a department responsible for the collection of data.
- Familiarize yourself with the National Institute for Clinical Excellence (NICE), its function and the guidance documents published. There is an excellent website (www.nice.org.uk). NICE has reviewed therapies for several long-term medical conditions and produced guidance. Register with NICE to receive all its guidance documents, which will give you an updated insight into current evidence-based guidelines.
- Collect any examples of changes to practice that result from a review of clinical data.

An example of a change to practice

- National guidelines suggest that clinically effective surgery should be performed within 24 hours for fractured necks of femurs. Bottlenecks in the patient journey resulted in an unacceptable pre-operative delay. Process redesign took place and a team of dedicated trauma nurses was appointed.

Clinical effectiveness

Clinical effectiveness is the process of ensuring that patient care is of the highest standard and is evidence based against current best practice. This can be broken into three steps:

- gathering and analysing the relevant evidence

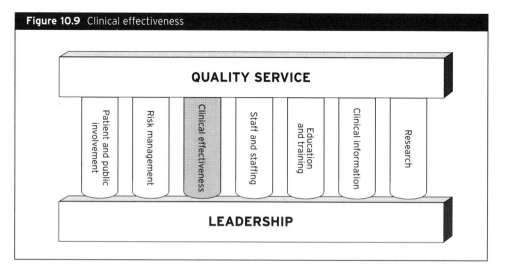

Figure 10.9 Clinical effectiveness

- analysing the findings and translating it to local implementation within the service
- evaluation of the implementation.

This evidence can be formally identified through clinical audit or research, or as a result of benchmarking care against similar trusts. *The Essence of Care* is a national project for benchmarking, which enables evaluation of the fundamental components of essential nursing care (NHS Modernisation Agency and DoH, 2003b).

Patient care should also be guided by national frameworks such as NICE guidelines, National Service Frameworks (NSFs) and results of external assessments such as those carried out by the Commission for Health Improvement (CHI). In addition, guidance from professional bodies such as the NMC or RCN Rheumatology Forum should be taken into account.

Pillar: research and audit

This section focuses on clinical audit, an often under-represented area within clinical care. Discussions on research issues are included in Chapter 5.

Clinical audit is a method of systematically reviewing clinical practice (e.g a review of prescribing appropriate pharmaceutical therapy to patients with osteoporosis) or the processes for delivering a service (e.g a review of patient waiting times in a rheumatology assessment clinic) by comparing *actual practice* with *agreed best practice*.

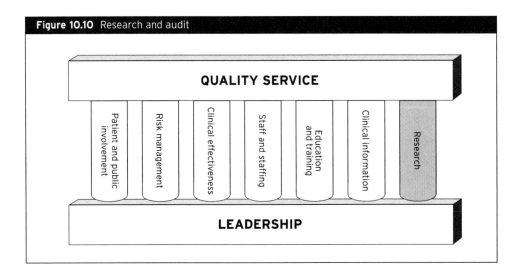

Figure 10.10 Research and audit

QUALITY SERVICE

Patient and public involvement · Risk management · Clinical effectiveness · Staff and staffing · Education and training · Clinical information · Research

LEADERSHIP

How is 'best practice' defined?

The 'gold standard' for practice or service provision can be determined in a variety of ways. Often the evidence base for best practice has been clearly described in the form of guidelines, appraisals or service frameworks issued by professional bodies such as the RCN or via national organizations (e.g. the National Osteoporosis Foundation). Nationally agreed guidelines or practice standards should be used as the basis of the audit, where they exist.

Discreet guidelines are not available for all areas of practice; instead it might be more appropriate to describe current practice against locally defined best practice.

Locally agreed standards are derived from expert opinion and inter-pretation of the current best research evidence. Typically, the available research is reviewed for a given treatment (e.g. pain management in arthritis) and local standards are formulated in light of the research evidence. It is important that all relevant professional groups are involved in the development of the standards, as lack of inclusiveness is a frequently quoted reason why changes to practice do not occur.

Background to clinical audit

Clinical audit was introduced in the late 1980s to review standards of clinical care and service provision. It is a key component of the quality improvement cycle and fundamental to the delivery of services within a clinical governance framework.

NICE defines clinical audit as 'a quality improvement process that seeks to improve patient care and *outcomes* through systematic review of care against explicit *criteria* and the implementation of change' (NICE, 2002b).

An audit project does need not be complex. Any section/process of a protocol, guideline, integrated care pathway or other documentation can be audited.

Practical steps

How to start an audit project:

- Remember the leadership qualities needed to implement a project/change or additional workload to the department. In addition, ensure that the wider healthcare team (e.g. healthcare assistants) is encouraged to participate in the audit process, building in a commitment to the project.
- Consult with colleagues. Prioritize clinical topics, as audit activity can be time-consuming and costly. Choose a topic that explores a high profile quality issue (e.g. patient complaints or high complication rates) or is concerned with high cost or risk to staff or users. Topics that focus on these key issues are more likely to be supported.

- Most NHS organizations have an audit department to support audit project design and it is worth visiting them. The name of the department can vary (e.g. clinical audit, clinical effectiveness, clinical governance support unit, clinical informatics, etc.), but they will be able to provide guidance and support. Depending on the audit planned, the lead nurse or doctor may need to endorse the project before it commences. The audit team can assist with the design of standards, literature reviews, data collection tools, analysis techniques and report writing. They will also be able to help with the dissemination of the audit results and action plans to change practice.
- Collect the audit data and present the findings. Collecting the data can be time-consuming. It is important to plan the audit carefully and allow enough time to complete the project.
- Change management – this is by far the most challenging aspect of the audit cycle. The success of implementing the identified needs for change will rely on collaborative working and enthusiasm from all members of the team. Additional resources may be required, so ensure that managers and commissioners are involved in the review process.
- Re-audit – closing the loop. This phase of the audit project is sometimes overlooked. However, reviewing practice following practice or service redesign is a useful way of comparing previous performance with current practice. Without regular review, performance can slip.

Examples of changes to practice

The rheumatology unit staff performed a documentation audit to review their integrated care pathway. This audit resulted in the following:

- Areas of the pathway demonstrated poor documentation and this led to further educational initiatives to demonstrate the value of record keeping.
- It raised awareness of the value of audit to all members of the team and added to their professional development, encouraging them to carry out more audit projects.

Conclusions

This chapter has discussed the key issues that will help to promote quality improvements in the provision of healthcare. Nurses are now at the forefront of developments and need to ensure they make an active contribution in the drive to establish a sound clinical governance structure. Failure to use these opportunities and recognize their value would be a retrograde step.

However, there are a number of factors to consider in the development of quality frameworks to protect the public and NHS staff. As this chapter has highlighted, the commitment of individual members of the team and their recognition of their role within a team are essential components for both effective leadershhip and clinical governance. The positive attributes and commitment of leaders within the organization to support teams are imperative. To develop a strong and useful approach to supporting clinical governance it can sometimes be useful to develop evidence folders reflecting each of the seven pillars discussed in this chapter. Document evidence and collate relevant data as an ongoing process in the implementation of quality improvements. It will certainly make any CHI review much easier!

The reality of clinical governance is that it brings the organization, managers and clinical staff together to improve the safety and quality of healthcare provision. The challenge for all healthcare professionals will be to meet these constantly changing agendas while keeping the patient as the focus.

Chapter 11

The patient's perspective

Ailsa Bosworth, John Skinner and Natalie Williams

Introduction

As nurses, the key driver and the most rewarding aspect of the role is that of providing clinical care by understanding and supporting the needs of the individual. Every nurse knows that one of the most powerful ways of understanding a disease is to look at the consequences of the disease from the patient's perspective. Health providers are increasingly aware of the need to recognize the expectations of the patient, not only to improve patient satisfaction but also for better health outcomes, more effective use of resources and appropriate management of clinical risk.

There are an increasing number of initiatives to highlight the patient's agenda, with health policies beginning to focus on addressing the 'patient's journey through healthcare' (DoH, 2001b). These issues do not come as a surprise for nurses, who have often been criticized for researching the *qualitative* rather than *quantitative* issues related to care. Yet qualitative research examining the patient's perspective and experiences provides rich and sometimes disappointing or distressing facts about failures in the provision of care. There are many excellent papers that highlight the needs of patients with long-term medical conditions (Holman and Lorig, 2000; Ryan et al., 2003). Nurses should read such papers related to their specific area of interest to capture the expectations and needs of the patient group that they care for.

It must be recognized that it is not always easy for patients to express their disappointment and needs openly, in a confident manner, although we may strive to enhance their ability to do exactly this. The difficulty in 'voicing' a view can be compounded by the fact that chronic disease management requires a long-term therapeutic relationship. Patients may fear that making their views known will 'threaten' that relationship, and ultimately their access to care (Oliver, 2001). This all sounds very harsh and negative, yet it is essential to remember that things are not always as they might seem. We can be made only too well aware of this issue when we have to cross over to the other side of the fence ourselves, and become a patient: despite all the best intentions it can be a very disempowering experience.

The 'illness trajectory' is a term used to describe the long and varied path that each one of us may experience when diagnosed with a long-term chronic disease (Charmaz, 1983; Corbin and Strauss, 1988; Kleinman, 1988; Gerhardt, 1990). It will be of value to review the psychological aspects of health and illness discussed in Chapter 4 before or after reading this chapter. The reader should reflect on:

- coping strategies
- health belief models
- loss of self – grief, loss and bereavement
- theory of reasoned action
- mastery and locus of control and self-efficacy.

It will then be valuable to review how these theoretical models impact on:

- patient choice
- informed consent
- concordance
- empowerment.

It is a pleasure to be able to include three individual stories about the consequences of coping with a chronic disease. The headings are chosen by each contributor and highlight their own perspective on their arthritis. Each one of these accounts is unique and highlights the need to be vigilant and aware of the individual's perspective in coming to terms with their disease.

Case study 1

My life with RA

I developed rheumatoid arthritis (RA) at the age of 31. Initially, I attributed the start of my disease to a bad fall that set off some back pain problems, interesting really when you know my family history that it never occurred to me I might be vulnerable to having RA! My father had severe RA and ankylosing spondylitis before I was born. He died aged 62 years, his disease having had a significant effect on his life and hastening his death. Sadly, despite his love for us, his disease, combined with an inability to truly express his emotions, has had an affect on the lives of both my brother and me, and also influenced the way I managed my disease with my husband and daughter.

At 31, I noticed that my right knee was swollen and a bit painful. I was married, commuting to London daily for work and had been trying to get pregnant for about four years.

I think I struggled on with this situation for the best part of 6–9 months before my boss finally got quite angry with me for not doing anything about it and sent me round the corner to see his doctor. The diagnosis was fairly swift – non-specific, seronegative polyarthritis. I found myself in hospital having fluid removed, the joint injected with steroid and my leg put in a light plaster cast for a week.

I didn't know that RA can reduce your fertility, so it was quite something to discover shortly afterwards that I was pregnant! You won't be surprised to hear that the RA improved considerably while I was pregnant! Anna was born and a few weeks after the birth, the RA returned with a vengeance.

Coping with a new baby is hard work enough without the added problem of RA. The fact that I had a high-powered job and that I could justify having a nanny had some advantages; the nanny could do all the difficult tasks for Anna but I had the joy of holding and playing with her. However, I did go through lots of difficult times with operations and struggling to rehabilitate. Over the years, with all the operations I have experienced, it is interesting to note that a common trait among surgeons is their failure to prepare people for what lies ahead after operations. So that first operation came as a bit of shock, when I realized the programme of rehabilitation that lay ahead.

The next few years followed with my attempts to stay at work, and just when one joint improved others played up. I had so many reviews, joint injections and different drugs to attempt to control my arthritis. I hated those joint injections; God, they were painful! The saving grace of all this was that I had a wonderful boss who supported me throughout maternity leave and then one hospitalization after another. It was so hard, as the challenge of my job and all the potential I could realize was tempered with the need to give in to one intervention after another.

I spent a lot of time sitting in rheumatology clinic waiting areas. I developed side effects to many of my treatments, and went through a range of other difficult tasks, such as learning to work with a splint on my left leg. To me the frustration was the time some things took to resolve. I had felt seriously ill and the culprit was my anti-inflammatory – but it took a year to pinpoint the cause. What a waste of a year. I did feel angry and over time I lost confidence in the consultant caring for me. This came to a head when I challenged a decision for a further synovectomy. I asked if I could seek a second opinion and found myself being ejected from the consultant's office in a most upsetting way and went home in tears at my wit's end. Anna was three and a half, my marriage was falling apart, I was trying to manage my busy job and all in all I was pretty low.

I would have so loved to have the opportunity to speak to a specialist rheumatology nurse or have access to the kind of multidiscliplinary team approach that is available in many centres now. A significant issue when you have a lifelong disease is that it is vital to like and respect your consultant because you're going to be working together for a very long time. I needed to develop a trusting relationship that would provide an opportunity to have an open discussion. I felt nobody understood my personal situation and was prepared to work with me to help me cope with my disease.

As sometimes happens, a chance meeting with a friend who had medical contacts led to my referral to a new consultant. I was put onto prednisolone, which made such a huge difference to the pain. I felt my life had been saved. I can remember the first day of being on steroids. I was flying to Germany for an exhibition and was dreading it. The long day and the difficulty standing and walking were a nightmare. However, that day I can remember the elation of walking down the steps of the plane like a grown up, not frantically holding onto the handrail, and facing the trip with a lot less dread than normal.

Things started to improve, I was now separated and had sorted Anna's little life out well. There was the minimum of disruption to her, and I had good childcare. I had a consultant I liked, respected and had confidence in, and I loved my job.

One more exciting step – I fell in love with Brian, the man who is now my husband, and we moved in together. He was also going through a divorce and, for the first time ever, I felt as though I had met my soul mate. My company had taken out private insurance for me. This was such a great relief – it meant I could see my consultant without having to wait! When you work long hours and have very little time, this makes a huge difference.

Over the years I had tried a range of disease-modifying anti-rheumatic drugs (DMARDs), all which failed to control the disease. Then I had an early menopause at age 40, having been on methotrexate injections. Yet another challenge!

There seemed to follow a roller coaster of events, with more operations on my hands, my career under threat with the firm having to go into voluntary liquidation, financial difficulties as a result and then an awful tragedy for my partner, whose son died while on holiday in India.

The emotional stress definitely affected my RA and for quite a long period I would have to spend one or two mornings a week in bed in order to be able to partially function the rest of the time. My hands and wrists were painful, making daily life difficult, when I suddenly had to have an emergency tendon repair. Again with no time to prepare myself I was back to a frustrating recovery time. I couldn't do very much for myself with only one semi-functional hand, and I couldn't drive.

I'm not very good at being dependent on others and I also find it difficult to wait for something to be done for me. Having to have help washing and dressing, going to the loo, etc., is not good news and have you ever tried wiping your bum with the wrong hand? A second operation on the other hand swiftly followed. However, after that recovery, the pain again became extreme and I became unable to lift anything, open anything, do up zips and buttons, etc.

Each time I recovered from one hurdle and learnt to readjust, another hurdle was put straight in front of me. I had to go through two wrist fusions, but they were worth doing.

My life with RA

I may have lost some function, but I also lost the pain. But the hurdles kept coming. My neck was the next bit that started to give major problems. The pain used to root me to the ground, but most of all it was very frightening as it felt a serious threat – would I suddenly become paralysed? My right hip needed to be replaced too, but they refused to operate until my neck was sorted out. Now I was busy stacking up the hurdles rather than spacing them out. I was so very frightened of the neck operation, more than any other operation I had been through. To make matters worse, I knew my hair would be cut. Oh the vanity of we women! The surgeon was great and managed to ensure the hair was cut in a way that it didn't show; with all that I had gone through these little attentions to my personal needs were greatly appreciated.

My husband has been fantastic and, although he would never have believed himself capable of being a carer, has become one in all senses of the word. I rely on him for so many things. On a positive note, he learnt to become a very good cook during this period. We still had a live-in mother's help who looked after Anna, taking her to and collecting her from school and doing the housework. This meant that her life (and therefore Brian's) was not disrupted every time I went into hospital. Having said that, she used to get very upset when I went in and always said to me on the day I was admitted, usually with tears running down her face, 'You're not going to die are you mummy?' I always involved Anna in my disease in a way that my mother and father had never done with me. In those days it was felt that children should be shielded from illness and anything difficult or unpleasant. I think that now Anna, at age 20, is a more sensitive and caring person to the problems others face.

After the neck surgery, I was tearful coming home. It is frightening how quickly you can become institutionalized. I felt safe in hospital with a nurse at the end of a buzzer, but at home I would be on my own while Brian was at work, and I was scared.

The neck improved for a time and I was able to have my hip replacement done the following April. Everyone said to me that my hip operation would be a doddle compared to my neck, so I was mildly surprised to wake up from the anaesthetic and think to myself,' God, this is so painful I don't feel as though I shall ever be able to walk again!' Somehow you get past these things and of course by the time I left hospital I could walk with crutches and even get up and down stairs. The hip operation has been very successful and it was such a relief to get rid of that grinding pain.

A few months passed and I was getting more pain in my neck again and a certain clicking noise on movement. I was x-rayed and it seemed that the bone graft had not taken, although the nuts and bolts were still in place! I had been worried that a screw was coming loose! My bone tissue was in poor condition due to the osteoporosis. I needed another operation, this time going in through the front of my neck and taking a piece of bone from my hip. He explained it was a bit like shoring up a crumbling wall. Nice analogy!

I was in tears. The thought of having to go through the neck operation again filled me with dread. This time I would have a horrible scar across the front of my neck too. It was all too much and I didn't want to know. I suppose I went into a kind of denial for a little while, but I am a realist if nothing else and it wasn't long before I had come to terms with the prospect of a second operation. At the end of the day I wanted to get rid of the pain. It was around this time that research trials were about to start with infliximab and my consultant referred me for consideration. It was a long process and everyone felt I would have a better chance with my neck operation if I had some treatment beforehand.

I started on anti-TNF treatment (infliximab) in February 2000. Within an hour and a half of having my first infusion I felt an improvement in my pain and stiffness. My quality of life was dramatically improved almost overnight! I could work for 8 hours, come home and, instead of collapsing unable to do anything more, could actually cook dinner! Amazing!

But of course, there was the second neck operation, including a bone graft taken from my hip, waiting for me. The surgeon was pleased with the outcome of the operation and although I continue to get neck/head pain on a daily basis, it is not as severe and I can live with it.

After my fourth and last infusion on the pre-licence trial of infliximab, I was told that, even though the drug had just obtained its licence in the UK, I would not be able to continue to have it. 'What?', I said. 'You cannot be serious!', to quote a certain famous tennis player. I fought a battle with everyone who would listen. My GP was very supportive writing to the primary care groups (PCG) and the health authority. My MP wrote to Alan Milburn (the then Secretary of State for Health) on my behalf. I spoke to a number of people on the committee evaluating anti-TNF treatment within my health authority. Everyone said 'no' to being able to obtain the treatment.

I simply wasn't prepared to accept this and finally, in desperation, wrote to the drug company. Initially I had no response so I wrote again. During this period of about six months I went rapidly downhill again, having several flares which simply made me more determined that I would not continue to feel like this when I knew I could feel a lot better! Just before Christmas 2000, I had a call from the drug company to say that they were prepared to supply the drug on 'compassionate' grounds. It was the best Christmas present I could have wished for.

It was this experience that gave birth to NRAS, the National Rheumatoid Arthritis Society, but that's another story.

The future?

That's a difficult one. A big step recently has been that of buying a wheelchair – it took quite some coming to terms with. You can feel very vulnerable and alone in a wheelchair. I watched a young woman pushing herself along a busy high street recently and thought how confident she looked. In spite of all that I have said, there is a small part of me that is quite terrified at the thought of having to manage in a wheelchair on my own.

I love my life in spite of the RA and the problems I face on a daily basis. I love my family, my friends, colleagues and my two jobs. But I am so fearful of anything happening to my husband because I am so reliant on him, and I don't want to be a burden, particularly to my daughter. I want them to enjoy life without having to worry about me. But as you may have ready guessed, I am a fighter and I shall continue to find ways of enjoying myself and also of improving the support and information that people with RA need.

The man and arthritis

This was a proud, fit, strong, macho, chauvinistic independent male – and proud of it! That was nearly five years ago – what happened then, almost overnight, was to change my life forever. I live on my own, I have always been fiercely independent and asking for help has never been on option – big boys don't cry, moan or complain!

Everything I do is affected by RA, my whole life revolves around it. This may sound pretty awful, but it's not, it's amazing how you adapt to new circumstances, and how what was a crisis at the beginning now becomes the norm. Though my arthritis is under control, it is always niggling away to remind me to adjust and pace myself. Apart from the occasional flare-up, my quality of life has become very good, but it is different from 'pre-arthritis days'. I become very tired every day and therefore need to be 'careful'. But this man has never been 'careful' in his life! I have always lived life in the fast lane, taking risks in business or in anything else has always excited me. I was a racing driver for 25 years and racing drivers don't drive 'carefully'! That is a contradiction in terms. I still work too long in the garden – up the ladders, cleaning out the gutters, etc. – and so pay the penalty. But I personally believe it is unwise to completely change your character just because of an illness, so some sort of compromise has to be found. Before detailing my experiences of arthritis it may be helpful to explain the character of this man, a brief potted history and where I was at the time my arthritis broke out.

If I had to describe myself in two words, I would say I am a 'shy extrovert'. Shyness has always plagued me and still does, and before my arthritis I always enjoyed the chance to be an extrovert!

At a very early age I was diagnosed with a lung disease called bronchiectasis, not good if you were, as I was, born in the smoke-laden city of Birmingham. Whether this condition was the result of whooping cough or pneumonia, I am not quite sure, but I had a constant cough throughout my childhood, difficulty in breathing and sleeping and always producing a lot of sputum. I was constantly described as a 'poorly child'. I was then and still am susceptible to infection. I was in and out of hospital with pneumonia and bronchitis; many bronchoscopies were carried out up until I was about 16. There, at an early age, I learnt to trust and enjoy hospitals. At the age of ten, half of my left lung was removed – a big operation in 1953! I remember the first two weeks in a dirty tent. The only things in focus were the hands and forearms as they thrust at me through the flaps of the oxygen tent – that was my little world.

I have always been happiest and most comfortable on my own. Not surprising, when I rarely went to primary school. I remember missing school for a whole year because I was so poorly. I missed a lot of education and hated being bottom of the class. I left school at 15 with nothing and a very poor education. I had always hoped to be a doctor – having been weaned on it! My career did improve with determination on my part and evening classes, gradually achieving a place at university and then ultimately qualifying as an architect. I loved amateur dramatics and finally gained an audition at the Old Vic theatre, but part of my audition involved catching a ball while reciting Shakespeare – needless to say I quickly became breathless and was dismissed. Yet another bitter pill. In the meantime, I went back to the routine work of an architect. Eventually a career opportunity came for me to take up racing driving and then run my own motor business – well why not? An occupation lying fully prone, on my back, doing very little in the fresh air – and not getting out of breath – has always appealed to me! Looking back I was very lucky to have a good marriage and two wonderful children. But, in 1983, my son Laurence, aged 17, died of a brain tumour. My whole world fell apart – he was my best mate, he came to every race meeting, we had always done everything together. While grieving his loss, my marriage quickly deteriorated and divorce followed without me really noticing. My wife left to remarry, taking my daughter with her. I was back to the lonely days of childhood. I consoled myself that after this disastrous period in my life nothing would ever be as bad – well arthritis got pretty close! I coped quite philosophically with a serious accident that ended my racing career, though I was already past my 'sell by date'.

I have carried too much baggage and emotion around. I have not found it easy to enter a relationship since my divorce. I have put a protective wall around myself. On reflection, perhaps I have always had this protective wall about me since childhood. So, I found my dream home in Devon, an abundance of gorgeous air to breath, acres and acres of garden to play in. I was content, happy and very much on my own, when after six months, and at the age of 55, the diagnosis of arthritis was probably the final straw that broke the camel's back!

Rheumatoid arthritis reduced me very quickly to a cabbage – this was not going to do my 'street cred' any good whatsoever! Flirting, dancing, weekends away – just being a normal competitive bachelor was no longer an option – it hurt. The disappointment of not being able to live your life as you wished was one thing, but the pain from arthritis was terrible – the immobility was pretty bad and the boredom was horrible – so I learnt that you could:

- take tablets for the pain
- obtain equipment for the immobility
- learn to read and watch daytime television (for the first time in my life) to help with the boredom.

Everything OK then? Well nothing has ever beaten this man and I was confident and determined to successfully adjust to and cope with arthritis. WRONG!

I could not get my head around the depressed state I was sinking into. Information was difficult to take in and retain. I struggled for two years, physically and mentally, with arthritis, but even after the medication started to kick in and I became more mobile, with less pain, I still found the mental depression continued. Looking back, I am sure this was compounded by my past history; it brought back my childhood days and there were long hours to mull over the loss of my son - he would have been there for me. I had no visitors. My parents and daughter lived hundreds of miles away. The future looked very bleak indeed.

I remember with horror the nurses helping me with my toilet requirements - being fed in public like a 'baby'. These incidents were big and important issues for me. For a man who hadn't cried for as long as I can remember, I was now crying every day. I did not want to leave the house. I only went out to visit my doctor or hospital. Shopping for food was a nightmare! On many, many occasions I got to the shop, panicked and drove home with nothing. I couldn't answer the phone, and contact with anyone reduced me to tears. Basically, I didn't want anyone to see this pathetic so-called MAN. This was completely against my normal character. Of course, I had experienced pain before, I had been sad, upset and very hurt, but never had I experienced this sort of depression.

A big factor in my recovery from depression was joining a local support group for arthritis suffers. I had to be slowly cajoled into doing this - it was totally against my wishes. But it worked - it was a great tonic. I slowly gained confidence and became an active member and made some good friends. The education I received in the hospital has also been vital in my recovery, but all of this has to come 'at the right time'. Patients will be traumatized by arthritis and you will have to be patient before bombarding them with 'what you know is good for them'!

This sad story is now completely behind me - I had to accept help. I was lucky in that I received a great deal of caring assistance. It was a huge package of rehabilitation that got me out of that black hole. As I said at the beginning, arthritis was to change my life forever. I now look at life very differently, but then many experiences in life can have this effect. As I am today, I can now dance (albeit in small bursts). Weekends away - no problem. Flirting - I'm working on it!

The girl – Natalie

When I was first diagnosed I had no idea what to expect and no one really explained what rheumatoid arthritis was or how bad it could get. I used to get really sick of people telling me what to do, instead of asking what I wanted. I now have much more control over my treatment and even little things like having a book to keep blood results in make a big difference. Before, I had no idea why I was having monthly blood tests or what the drugs I was taking were doing. I was totally unprepared for the side effects that came with the medication, which were really severe and scared me and my parents.

In the space of a year I went from a very independent 14-year-old to someone who needed her mum to help her get dressed, and it seemed all people were doing was telling me what I couldn't do. I knew all too well what I could and couldn't do, what I really needed was someone to help me find other ways to achieve things, or to ask what I thought, or just to say 'it's up to you'. Things are very different now, and it's so nice not to dread my next hospital appointment.

It took me quite a while to adjust to having arthritis; it came on very quickly and I went from being in the school netball and hockey teams to not even doing PE. I'm not very good at talking about my feelings and felt quite alone at times. It's hard for other people to understand because they can't see anything wrong with you. Teenagers can be really bitchy, and if one day you're OK and the next you're limping then you start hearing comments about faking it flying around! I've always had good friends to support and stick up for me and there were times at school when I wouldn't have lasted the day without them. One of the hardest things about having arthritis is the amount of school or college you miss. The last two years at school I always seemed to be behind and could never quite catch up. I found it hard to ask for extra help, which I think had something to do with not wanting to stand out. I'm still not very good at talking to my lecturers about why I miss days at college and I don't think they really understand. It's hard to make people realize that there's more to it than just having stiff joints, that you can feel really tired and if your joints are bad then you can feel quite ill too. I didn't see anyone except a consultant for the first two years and, looking back, it would probably have made things much easier if there had been someone else to talk to.

I have always ridden horses and got my first horse about four months before I was diagnosed. Even when I felt really bad I never stopped riding, and sometimes it was the only time I could do everything my friends did. At one hospital appointment I was told I shouldn't ride anymore and definitely not more than once a fortnight. It was much worse than being told I had arthritis and I was so upset. I didn't ride for two weeks and then after a big argument with my parents I started again and haven't stopped since. I hated the way someone who I didn't even know could make a snap decision about something so important to me. I used to be completely intimidated during hospital appointments and it didn't help that it was never me who was being talked to - it was always my parents. I can remember being poked and prodded while being talked about like I wasn't there. I'm glad to say things are now 100% better, mainly because I know there's always someone to talk to if I need it. I've always had male consultants, which made it even harder to talk openly, especially at 14. I think having female nurses is really important, because some things you just don't feel comfortable talking about with a man. I find it much easier to talk to women and when you're feeling really bad you need someone to talk to, especially because I'm not very good at talking about things with my family.

I think the most important thing is feeling in control and you can't feel in control if you're being told all the time rather than being asked. At 14 you hate being told what to do anyway and it was really hard to have limitations put on what I could do. Now the disease is much more under control and I try not to let having arthritis stop me doing anything. And if there's something I can't do then at least it's my choice, which makes all the difference. That doesn't mean that I don't have bad days, but at least now I don't feel alone. Sometimes I get scared about what the future will hold. It can be hard, because the clinics I attend often have people there who are much worse than me, who are in a wheelchair and can't use their hands. There are lots of uncertainties, like whether the medication will continue to work, or what will happen if I want to have children, or whether I'll be able to travel after uni. Things that I never thought about a few years ago, but which now I seem to spend more and more time thinking about.

Conclusions

These stories bring out a number of issues that, in theory, we are all aware of when caring for individuals who have a chronic disease. The uniqueness of each story reflects the immensely complex aspects of providing appropriate support and information based on the individual's specific needs. The nurse's skill in having an open and mutually respectful relationship, taking the time to recognize the patient's perspective and individual specific needs, is an area of immense importance. The therapeutic relationship needs to develop over time and the patient's illness experience.

It may also be useful at the end of this chapter to reflect on and review the theoretical concepts related to coping with a chronic illness. For a detailed discussion, refer to Chapter 4, Ryan et al. (1996), Hill (1998) and Further reading on page 273.

Chapter 12

Working with organizations

Janet Cushnaghan, Janice Mooney, David GI Scott and Jane Tadman

Introduction

This chapter has been prepared with contributions from some of the key representatives within the speciality of rheumatology. There are similar networks within other areas of chronic disease management.

It is essential to recognize the value of patient and professional groups working together to improve care and maintain professional standards. Whatever the specialist area, there will be organizations that will either support the patient group or work with healthcare professionals to support the needs of patients and the overall strategic development of the service. These groups can be effective in raising standards, as well as working as a combined force in lobbying healthcare providers and governing bodies to recognize the needs of the patients.

An example of collaborative working is that of the Arthritis and Musculoskeletal Alliance (ARMA). This umbrella organization brings together primary and secondary care physicians, and patient groups representing a wide range of musculoskeletal diseases (including Arthritis Research Campaign (**arc**), Arthritis Care, Lady Hoare Trust for Physically Disabled Children, Lupus UK, National Ankylosing Spondylitis Society, National Rheumatoid Arthritis Society and many more). Professional groups include the Royal College of Nursing (RCN), British Society for Rheumatology (BSR), British Healthcare Professionals in Rheumatology (BHPR), British Orthopaedic Association (BOA) and British Paediatric Rheumatology Group (BPRG) to mention just a few.

It is hoped that this chapter will highlight the value of working across organizational boundaries with other professional and patient groups to raise awareness and achieve the optimum in knowledge and expertise. As practitioners working within a specific area of healthcare, the excellent work undertaken within your own field of practice can have a rewarding impact locally. However, cascading knowledge and expertise to develop new ways of working or simply to formalize recognized standards of good practice can be enhanced when working collaboratively with other professional bodies on the 'bigger picture'. This chapter aims to provide:

- an understanding of the nature and variety of organizations supporting improvements in standards of care, using a rheumatology example
- a brief overview of the collaborative working and support that can be provided working together
- examples of how nurses can effect change working at a national level.

The Arthritis Research Campaign (arc), by Jane Tadman, arc press officer

For the past few years, rheumatology nurse practitioners have been leading the field as one of the fastest-growing specialties in the nursing profession. Despite this fact, some senior nurses working in these extended roles – often running outpatient clinics and working closely with rheumatologists – became increasingly frustrated by the lack of opportunity to develop a career pathway and a chance to carry out clinical research.

It was very much in response to this sense of frustration that the Arthritis Research Campaign (arc), the UK's fourth biggest medical research charity, began to consider how best to develop this career pathway for experienced rheumatology nurses.

An extensive survey conducted by the charity's education subcommittee revealed widespread support for strengthening the career structure of allied healthcare professionals working in rheumatology through the creation of academic posts within rheumatology rather than nursing departments. As a result, arc set up a pilot scheme of five-year lecturer and senior lecturer posts in academic nursing and for other allied health professionals.

The only criteria for applying were the presence of an academic department linked to a school of nursing actively involved in research, and protected research time for the post-holder and an appropriate research programme. Posts were awarded only where there was strong commitment from the university to continue them at the end of five years.

The Arthritis Research Campaign (arc) went on to pump more than £1 million into five lectureships – a hefty financial commitment as well as a change of direction for a charity that had previously concentrated its resources on funding basic science in university medical schools and clinical research in rheumatology departments, but not nurse-led work.

Three of the posts awarded went to senior nurses, the other two to an academic physiotherapist and an academic podiatrist. All three nursing post-holders are already combining running clinics with clinical research and teaching responsibilities.

The new posts have been well received by the rheumatology nursing community. Sarah Ryan, now the UK's first rheumatology nurse consultant at Haywood Hospital in Stoke on Trent, said: 'arc has been visionary in developing an academic career structure for health professionals (including nurses, physiotherapists and podiatrists) who wish to pursue education and research interests, with the creation of the lectureships. The combination of arc's new commitment and the government's creation of the first nurse consultant posts are aimed at reducing the number of senior nurses leaving the profession. These initiatives should ensure that heath professionals can utilize their skills appropriately in clinical care and research settings, with the shared goal of improving patient outcome.'

What has been achieved by these nursing lecturers so far?

Dr Jackie Hill, a leading nurse practitioner in Leeds who has been active in supporting opportunities to expand and advance the role of the nurse over many years, became an arc senior lecturer in rheumatology nursing in 2000.

Partly as a result of the arc endowment to Dr Hill, a new Academic and Clinical Unit of Musculoskeletal Nursing (ACUMeN) was launched in March 2003 to provide an academic focus for rheumatology nurses throughout Yorkshire. ACUMeN is a collaboration of the University of Leeds' School for Healthcare Studies, the Academic Unit of Musculoskeletal Disease and Leeds Teaching Hospitals Trust, and recognizes that rheumatology nurses have an important role to play in improving patient care and treatment by carrying out clinical research.

Dr Hill, who is a co-director of ACUMeN, explains: 'The aim of the unit is to generate, disseminate and apply knowledge in order to improve practice and patient outcomes with rheumatology nursing. Our work will be firmly rooted in practice.'

ACUMeN will also provide an opportunity for clinically and university-based nurses to collaborate in developing the evidence base that is needed to provide high-quality patient care, as well as enhancing nurses' professional development and opening up new career pathways in research.

Research funded by arc and carried out by Dr Hill has already established that arthritis patients attending outpatient clinics run by senior nurses do better than those attending clinics run by junior doctors, and that nurses need more training to help them deal with patients with sexual problems associated with rheumatoid arthritis.

Dr Sarah Hewlett, a former clinical nurse manager at Bristol Royal Infirmary, became an arc senior lecturer in rheumatology (health professions) in 2001. While running a nurse specialist clinic once a week, Dr Hewlett is also heavily involved in a great deal of collaborative research, much of this involving NHS Research and Development. 'The theme of our programme is to try and find out what issues are important to patients, and to see if we can measure them in terms of impact,' she explains. 'Then we will try and put these two things together and look at what health professionals are doing for patients. It's very practical work.'

Meanwhile Dr Hewlett is, thanks to arc funding, carrying out a national survey to find out if nurses, physiotherapists and occupational therapists learn enough about rheumatology during their training. This is against a backdrop of increasing difficulties in filling specialist rheumatology health professional posts.

In addition, Dr Hewlett is studying fatigue in rheumatoid arthritis using focus groups: how to define it, measure it and treat it, as well as looking at the best ways to deliver self-management strategies.

The third arc lecturer in rheumatology nursing, Candy McCabe, based at the Royal National Hospital for Rheumatic Diseases in Bath, is undertaking research as part of a her PhD. She is studying rheumatological pain, in particular fibromyalgia and complex regional pain syndrome or reflex sympathetic dystrophy. Mrs McCabe holds two clinics a week, one nurse specialist clinic and the other a pain clinic.

It is still early days for these lectureships, and arc is currently consulting widely to look at the means of enhancing academic research and the role of allied health professionals. However, there seems little doubt that the lectureships have already acted as a catalyst for new developments in the careers of senior rheumatology nurses, and are helping to develop better clinical care and patient management – which is excellent news for arthritis patients as well as senior nurses themselves.

The Royal College of Nursing

The Royal College of Nursing (RCN) mission statement is that: 'The RCN represents nurses and nursing, promotes excellence in practice and shapes health policies.' This is achieved by lobbying government for changes in policy, recognizing the contribution of nurses and aiding their development professionally.

Nurses joining the RCN can access speciality groups (forums). Each forum consists of a steering committee made up of nurses who have been elected to represent the speciality group. Their post is unpaid and the type of work they undertake will vary according to the needs of their group. The Chair of the RCN Rheumatology Forum provides an overview below.

Whatever your specialist area of interest it is likely that there will be at least two to three forums that may be useful for you to join. You can select the forums you wish to join. The Rheumatology Forum work highlights similar work in other specialist areas of interest.

The Royal College of Nursing Rheumatology Forum, by Janice Mooney, Chair

Vicky Stephenson established the Royal College of Nursing Rheumatology Forum (RCNRF) in March 1981. Initially, the Forum was set up to provide advice and support to promote the role of nurses working in the speciality of rheumatology. The Forum has changed over time, extending development in a range of ways according to national policies, the needs of nurses and the best ways of supporting excellence in care.

Aims and objectives of the Forum

The RCNRF aims to represent and promote the vital role of the nurse in caring for patients who have a rheumatic disease in any care setting. It is concerned with patient safety and ensuring that patients receive quality care. This may mean that the committee works on policy documents or gets involved in lobbying with patient groups, depending on current issues. It will campaign on a wide range of areas that impact on the nursing and patient care agenda relevant to daily practice. Committee work is challenging but often rewarding. It provides an opportunity to have a voice in government agendas and raise the profile of the speciality and the nurse working in it.

Does the Forum have a value to practitioners ?

It is likely that you will find contact with the Forum helpful if you have:
- recently been appointed to a specialist post in rheumatology
- taken on a new and different role

- found that you are now caring for rheumatology patients
- become involved in the assessment and management of patients receiving biologic agents
- felt isolated or wanted to know who to contact for specialist advice or knowledge
- want to access awards and bursaries that will aid in your professional development and improve patient care

What can you expect from becoming a Rheumatology Forum member?

One of the most popular benefits is that of a newsletter, distributed twice a year. It provides news on new courses and developments, feedback on national conferences, and an opportunity for members to write and contribute their views to Forum members. It offers information about a range of important educational events as well as the RCNRF annual conferences. The Forum conferences are organized by either a committee member or a Forum member, and we are extremely grateful for their support in this. The conferences are organized so that cost to the individual nurse is kept to a minimum, in order to encourage as many nurses as possible to attend.

In addition, the newsletter provides information on various bursaries and awards that are available to assist with attendance at conferences and study days. The RCNRF offers a bursary each year for a nurse to be able to attend the national rheumatology nursing conference, as well as other awards.

One innovative idea developed by the Forum is working with pharmaceutical companies. For example, Pharmacia (now Pfizer) provides a bursary that enables the recipient to attend the American College of Rheumatology annual conference. Awards such as these encourage nurses to recognize their value and gain confidence in implementing change. The award winner also gains experience in presenting, as they are often asked to inform others about their work, especially at the RCN National Conference. The rewards of attending an international conference will be felt by both the nurse and the patients, who reap the benefit of the nurse's newfound knowledge.

Forum members network with each other and access other nurses and healthcare professionals within the field for information and advice. This helps to guide the committee members on the issues that need developing to improve clinical care.

Are there specific roles within the committee?

Yes there are. The Forum committee is elected by the RCN membership and part of the committee's role is to develop guidelines and/or policies that are relevant and topical to nurses working in the speciality. The current Forum has developed specific roles for each member of the committee, which allows a fair division of labour as well as enabling links and expertise to develop in a specific aspect of Forum work. Committee members are currently allocated to:

- chair
- representative on ARMA and BSR committees
- newsletter editor
- website co-ordinator
- leadership
- strategic development
- policy and guidelines
- conference organizers and bursaries.

In addition to these roles, members will also be on working parties or committees (e.g. National Institute for Clinical Excellence (NICE), National Patient Safety Agency (NPSA) and Biologics Register (BR)) or supporting other members by sharing their workload.

One committee member is responsible for collation of our submissions of resolutions for debate at the Annual RCN Congress held in Harrogate. Examples of submission have included postcode prescribing, free prescriptions for rheumatology patients and funding to support the introduction of NICE-approved drugs. Events have also been organized at the National RCN Congress to raise awareness of musculoskeletal disease issues. In 2003, the Rheumatology Forum was joint organizer of a 'Forgotten Diseases' debate at Congress – encouraging nurses to recognize the needs of arthritis patients and raise active discussions and media coverage on the needs of musculoskeletal disease groups.

What power does the Forum have?

Acting as a professional group representing nurses in a particular speciality provides an opportunity to develop ideas and access key advice. It has the potential to influence in politically important arenas, as already highlighted; one such setting is the National RCN Congress. The power the Forum has at the National Congress is that of a formal voting allocation. The number of votes each forum has depends on the number of members registered with that forum. Each forum is allocated one vote per 1000 members who select the forum as their first choice.

Therefore to have a voting voice to represent our members' views and respond to the debates, it is important to have as many votes as possible. Unfortunately, the Forum currently has only one vote at congress and this significantly reduces the options in negotiating support and lobbying opportunities with other nursing forums to drive through key patient issues. As a member of the RCN, each person can elect to have up to three forums as part of their membership without additional charge. The enthusiasm and interest of Forum members add to the rewards of being a committee member.

The work of the committee frequently spills over into personal time so it is not a role for the faint-hearted! The following gives a flavour of the issues recently undertaken.

Guidance documents

- *Standards for Effective Practice and Audit in Rheumatology Nursing: Guidance for nurses* (RCN, 2001).
- *A Charter for Rheumatology Nursing* (RCN, 2000b).
- Various guidelines for disease-modifying drugs and intra-articular injections.
- *Guidance for Practitioners in the Assessment, Administration and Monitoring of Biologic Therapies for Inflammatory Arthritis* (RCN, 2003a).

Other work

- Organizing and running RCN rheumatology nursing conferences.
- Working on reviews and evidence for NICE and NPSA.
- Preparing for the annual RCN congress. This involves researching the most effective ways of raising key issues with politicians and congress members
- Raising awareness of the Forum.
- Preparing the content of the Forum newsletter for publication.
- Meetings with organizations or patient groups that wish to liaise with the Forum for support or advice.
- The development of an RCN Rheumatology Forum website.

And all in your spare time!

Preparing new documents is often achieved by setting up a working party, made up of a committee member and members of the Forum with particular expertise, or in other circumstances working with other groups from ARMA.

All the committee members act as a point of contact to provide support, information and advice to Forum members on issues in current practice. If a member phones the RCN they may be directed to a Forum member for specialist advice or put in contact with someone locally.

A fundamental role is that each committee member will act as an expert resource to RCN council members. This may take the form of providing advice on any major policy issues in rheumatology, commenting on consultation documents or dealing with media enquiries. It is usually the chair's responsibility to respond on behalf of the committee.

The RCN is asked to comment on a wide range of consultation documents that have an impact on rheumatology issues, and this includes patient care and nursing issues. The majority have a short timescale for response and require prompt action by the chair.

Two examples of consultation documents that the chair has responded to are the NICE submissions for cyclo-oxygenase (COX2) anti-inflammatory agents and the new biologic agent anakinra, for the treatment of rheumatoid arthritis. The chair responds to these documents on behalf of the RCN members. A more lengthy process was the submission to NICE on anti-TNFα drugs. The RCN Rheumatology Forum (in collaboration with other members of ARMA) responded to the submission for anti-TNFα therapies.

How can I become a committee member?

Once you are an RCN member you can submit your nomination to be elected as a committee member when there are notifications of elections. Vacancies for positions on the committee are advertised in the newsletter, RCN bulletins and mail shots. Be prepared for plenty of hard work and learning on your feet.

What are the challenges for the future?

The boundaries of nursing practice are continuously being extended, which has led to overlap of doctors' and nurses' roles. Nurses have developed their clinical practice with enhanced practice skills and strengthened educational and academic qualifications. The result is a plethora of nurse-led clinics where nurses are able to see and treat patients, sometimes supported by the use of protocols. New national initiatives such as walk-in centres and NHS Direct have seen the nurse become the first point of contact for patients. Nurses are now legally able to prescribe medicines as either an independent or a supplementary prescriber after completing a recognized course.

Clinical practice is forging ahead and, as nurses are taking on these new roles, responsibility and accountability for patient care are greater than ever before. Continued personal and professional development is the key for nursing to survive the radical reforms set out in *The New NHS: Modern, dependable* and *The NHS Plan* (DoH, 1997, 2000a). The future holds many opportunities and challenges, and to strengthen nurses' contribution to healthcare we must ' become leaders of change'.

The British Health Professionals in Rheumatology, by Janet Cushnaghan, President 2000–2001

The BHPR was established in 1985 to bring together all the disciplines of healthcare professionals whose major interest lay in the care of people with rheumatic diseases. For the first time in the UK there was a society encompassing all members of the multidisciplinary team involved in the management of rheumatic diseases.

The aims of the BHPR

- To encourage and emphasize the multidisciplinary approach to the care of people with rheumatic diseases.
- To provide a forum through which health professionals can exchange knowledge, skills and experience.
- To generate greater awareness of the contribution of health professionals.

Membership of the society is open to all healthcare professionals who wish to strengthen their involvement and education in rheumatology and to share their knowledge and expertise, or are simply new to the field and would welcome the opportunity to network with fellow professionals in the speciality. New members from overseas are particularly welcome. There are 'sister' organizations in many countries already and we have held joint meetings with some of these societies. This increases the circle for networking beyond the UK into the rheumatology community world-wide.

Disciplines represented in the membership include nurses, physiotherapists, occupational therapists, doctors, pharmacists, podiatrists, dieticians, psychologists and social workers. The society has strong links with other groups in the UK such as the BSR, RCNRF, National Association of Rheumatology Occupational Therapists (NAROT),

Rheumatic Care Association of Chartered Physiotherapists (RCACP) and the Podiatry Rheumatic Care Association (PRCA). In addition, we have representation on ARMA, arc, Arthritis Care, the National Electronic Library for Health and the arc/BSR Clinical Trials Collaboration. These links and BHPR representation in other groups ensure that the voice of healthcare professionals is reaching all parties concerned and members of the BHPR council are working with other groups, rather than being isolated and perhaps duplicating effort.

The governing body of the BHPR is the Council, consisting of eight officers: president, president elect or immediate past president, honorary secretary, honorary treasurer, communications officer, deputy honorary secretary, deputy honorary treasurer and deputy communications officer. The Council meets several times a year and is responsible for deciding the arrangements for all meetings and other business of BHPR and for determining its representatives to other bodies. All candidates for election to office require nomination by two ordinary members of the society. To be eligible for nomination as president, a candidate must have served on Council. Officers are elected at each Annual General Meeting and assume their duties on 1 January the following year. The BSR office provides administrative support for the BHPR.

A BHPR handbook is produced for members. The handbook not only has a list of members, to facilitate communicating with colleagues, but it also has a list of professionals who have agreed to being approached if members need advice. In addition, it includes a list of useful organizations for rheumatological conditions as well as general organizations.

Regular newsletters are circulated to members. They report on conferences and meetings as well as sharing members' work, and they also feature news articles, book reviews and a diary of events.

The BHPR is able to offer bursaries and prizes each year to members. Currently annual travel bursaries are offered to several members to attend courses or conferences or support for an educational visit, to another unit, for example. Each year the BHPR judges entries for a clinical prize, as well as acting on behalf of arc to judge a piece of research work. The winning entry is awarded the prestigious arc prize and silver medal.

Council constantly reviews the work of the BHPR. An example of new development is the addition of a poster prize at the annual spring conference. The BHPR evolves as the society grows and changes according to the needs of its members.

Currently the BHPR host two conferences a year. The spring meeting is combined with the BSR AGM, promoting clinical research. BHPR encourages abstract submission from the membership. Presentation is by poster or oral presentation and abstracts are published in *Rheumatology*.

Traditionally the autumn conference, including the AGM, has a clinical theme with guest speakers, workshops and even practical sessions. Special interest groups for rheumatoid arthritis, osteoporosis and connective tissue diseases started in 2002. Sessions are held at the spring meetings, and convenors of each special interest group invite guest presenters or chair general discussion on the topic concerned. In this way, people interested in particular topics can meet on an informal basis in smaller numbers than at plenary sessions, share ideas and start collaborative working.

The BHPR encourages its members to participate in research, and a number of members currently involved in research are available to offer help and advice to new researchers. BHPR provides a forum, via conferences, for work to be widely disseminated and debated.

As far as education is concerned, by providing a wide variety of topics at conferences and a valuable listing of courses, BHPR provides several avenues of professional development. The education of health professionals is promoted through representation on the arc education subcommittee, and the arc allied health professionals working group of the education subcommittee has been awarded a large research grant to develop an education structure for health professionals working in extended roles in rheumatology.

In conjunction with the BSR, BHPR is developing a new website, which will expand communication among members with discussion boards, news, features and conference listings. The sharing of information via the Internet is the way forward in this technological age and BHPR is proud to be part of it.

A personal perspective on the role of the nurse in rheumatology care, by Professor David GI Scott, President of the British Society for Rheumatology, 2002

The role of the nursing profession in caring for patients with arthritis is well established. Traditionally this has been on wards, when patients are brought in for care with flares of arthritis and for investigations of connective tissue disease. Nurses have also for many years supported traditional outpatient clinics with contributions to patient care and education. In some academic units, nurse practitioners began to develop. This was a different role, mainly monitoring patients during follow-up on second-line drugs, and early studies showed their effectiveness to be equal to (often better than) conventional doctor-led clinics (Hill et al., 1994; Hill, 1997). This was no great surprise, given the increased time nurse practitioners spend with patients (compared to doctors), and supported similar experiences in other disciplines, particularly diabetes and hypertension, where it is now recognized that nurses are more effective than doctors in this role.

The past decade, however, has seen a rapid expansion and a major change in the role of nurses and practitioners in rheumatology. Some of this reflects our increasing ability to intervene with the natural history of inflammatory arthritis and the use of more complex and more effective therapies. There is now an established pattern of nurse practitioner involvement in most rheumatology units throughout the country, such that the adage that 'every unit should have one' is now changed into 'every unit must have several'! In Norwich, for example, we have four nurse practitioners whose role has expanded to include education, monitoring, advice in primary care, assessment and some therapeutic interventions. This development initially took place in secondary care but increasingly now bridges the gap between primary and secondary care. For example, in Norwich, eight GP practices have visiting nurse practitioners from our unit undertaking clinics in the surgery or adjacent hospitals, and our nurse practitioners frequently advise GPs about clinical practice within the hospital setting and ease the transfer of patients between the two systems.

Audits have been undertaken to support the success of such developments and there is little doubt that patient care is hugely enhanced by these developments, with improved satisfaction, a reduction in travel, and greater continuity of care with more understanding and sympathetic practitioners (Mooney, 1999; Horrocks et al., 2002). It seems likely that such developments will continue in the future, particularly with the increasing recognition of expanded roles, such as prescribing and nurse/practitioner consultant posts. The opportunities will enable more independent roles that will continue to bridge the primary–secondary care interface.

The development of such specialization also supports educational aspirations of the professions. Almost all nurses now undergo undergraduate education and those involved in specialist nurse practitioner roles, such as rheumatology, are frequently involved in taking part in multidisciplinary Masters degree programmes, involving nurses, therapists, podiatrists and doctors. Their involvement is also strategically vital to undergraduate medical school programmes, such as the novel integrated course at the University of East Anglia.

Within the BSR, recognition of the role of nurse practitioners includes support for the infrastructure of the BHPR and their academic programme. At the BSR annual meetings, a significant numbers of doctors attend the BHPR programme, where one may find more clinically orientated presentations than in some of the scientific sessions. I hope in future that we will have even greater integration with BHPR presentations at the plenary session of the BSR. Perhaps full integration between BSR and BHPR is not far away. Just as scientists are included as full BSR members (with reduced subscriptions), so should BHPR members be; thus, we will have one broad church in the BSR inevitably, and at some stage a scientist or health professional as president – why not?

The above suggests a natural progression and integration of services that may be a few years away. I do, however, feel that we can look at the present situation to provide an ideal service for our patients, especially with the use of the new biologic agents and the enormous benefit that they have brought to our patients with inflammatory arthritis. This could occur in three settings:

- A hospital-based service will continue for complex patients, for diagnosis of patients and for inpatients, and this will probably be run, as now, with consultants, junior doctor support and nurse practitioner support for education and initial instigation of second-line therapy.
- The community units and community hospitals will further develop and there will be more independence for nurse practitioners to undertake their own clinics (with consultant advice), liaising with GPs.
- Within general practice itself I see nurse practitioners conducting clinics alongside GPs, giving advice in both directions and referring patients back to hospital where necessary.

The role of the different organizations in supporting such developments is complex. The RCN Forum may have a similar role to the Royal College of Physicians Joint Speciality Committee, with the College taking a broader role and supporting rheumatology as a speciality, but with the BSR providing the professional support for clinicians. Similarly, the RCN will provide advice and development for the nursing profession in general and the RCN Nursing Forum will be equivalent to the Joint Speciality Committee linking and liaising with the BHPR.

All of us need to collaborate more closely, linking with patient groups and with the research fraternity, such as arc. This we will, hopefully, continue to achieve through the developments of ARMA, which, although in its infancy, is the main political workforce that will support and advertise the enormous developments of our speciality in the future. We will, with luck, be able to have a national plan for arthritis in the UK, just as has been successfully launched in Wales, but this requires the collaboration and support of all health professions, patient groups and research organizations under the umbrella of ARMA. This we can do only if we develop the appropriate standards of care demanded by patients and ask organizations for the resources to deliver them. As always we need to act together.

Appendix 1

Chief Nursing Officer –
ten key roles for nurses in
The NHS Plan (DoH, 2000a)

- To order diagnostic investigations such as pathology tests and x-rays.
- To make and receive referrals direct to, for example, a therapist or pain consultant.
- To admit and discharge patients for specified conditions and within agreed protocols.
- To manage patient caseloads, e.g. for diabetes or rheumatology.
- To run clinics, e.g. for ophthalmology or dermatology.
- To prescribe medicines and treatments.
- To carry out a wide range of resuscitation procedures, including defibrillation.
- To perform minor surgery and outpatient procedures.
- To triage patients using the latest IT to the most appropriate health professionals.
- To take a lead in the way health services are organized and run.

Appendix 2

Website addresses

ACAS (personnel information)	www.acas.org.uk
AIMS2	www.qolid.org.uk
British Society for Rheumatology (guidelines)	www.rheumatology.org.uk
British Society for Rheumatology Biologics Register	www.arc.man.ac.uk
Clinical governance	www.doh.gov.uk/clinicalgovernance www.cgsupport.org
Clinical Governance Bulletin	www.rsmpress.co.uk/cgb.htm
Clinical Governance Information Team	www.nhsia.nhs.uk/phsmi/clinicalgovernance
Clinical Supervision (clinical supervision guidance)	www.clinical-supervision.com
Commission for Health Improvement (CHI)	www.chi.nhs.uk
Commission for Patient and Public Involvement in Health (CPPIH)	www.cppih.org.uk
Copyright	www.nfer-nelson.co.uk
Department of Health (policy documents and Chief Nursing Officer bulletins)	www.doh.gov.uk
Health Technology Assessment Systematic Reviews	www.hta.nhsweb.nhs.uk
Modernisation Agency (guides to improving patient care)	www.modern.nhs.uk/improvementguides

National Electronic Library for Health (evidence-based database)	www.nelh.nhs.uk
National Patient Safety Agency (a health authority to improve safe administration of treatments)	www.npsa.nhs.uk
NHS quality improvement Scotland	ww.nhsquality.org
Nursing & Midwifery Council (professional issues and regulation)	www.nmc.org.uk
Ombudsman	www.ombudsman.org.uk
Patient Information Sheets	www.arc.org.uk
RAQoL	galen@galen-research.com
Research governance	www.info.doh.gov.uk
RCN Library	www.rcn.org.uk
RCN Rheumatology Forum website/newsletter	www.rcn.org.uk
Royal College of Nursing (professional issues, information)	www.rcn.org.uk
SF-36	www.sf-36.org/copyright.shtml
Summary of Product Characteristics	www.medicines.org.uk

Databases to access

• AMED (Allied and Alternative Medicine)

• BNI (British Nursing Index)

• CINAHL (Cumulative Index, Nursing and Allied Health Lit)

• Cochrane Library (evidence-based healthcare)

• MEDLINE (medicine)

• PsychINFO (psychology)

Appendix 3

Useful addresses

Age Concern
Astral House
1268 London Road
London SW16 4ER
Tel: 020 8765 7200

Arthritis and the Musculoskeletal Alliance
41 Eagle Street
London WC1 4AR
Tel: 020 7841 5191

Arthritis Care
18 Stephenson Way
London NW1 2HD
Tel: 020 7380 6500

Arthritis Research Campaign
St Mary's Court
St Mary's Gate
Chesterfield
Derbyshire S41 7TD
Tel: 01246 558033

British Geriatric Society
31 St John's Square
London EC1M 4DN
Tel: 020 7608 1369

British Healthcare Professionals Allied to Rheumatology
c/o 41 Eagle Street
London WC1 4AR
Tel: 020 7242 3313

British Society for Rheumatology
41 Eagle Street
London WC1 4AR
Tel: 020 7242 3313

Chartered Society of Physiotherapy
14 Bedford Row
London WC1R 4ED
Tel: 020 7306 6666

The College of Occupational Therapists
106–114 Borough High Street
London SE1 1LB
Tel: 020 7357 6480

College of Osteopaths Practitioners Association
13 Furzehill Road
Borehamwood
Hertfordshire WD6 2DG
Tel: 020 8905 1937

Disabled Living Foundation
380–384 Harrow Road
London W9 2HU
Tel: 020 7289 6111

Institute of Orthopaedics
Royal National Orthopaedic
Hospital, 45–51 Bolsover Street
London W1W 5AQ
Tel: 020 7387 5070

National Ankylosing Spondylitis
Society
179 Mayfield
East Sussex TN20 6ZL
Tel: 01435 873527

National Back Pain Association
16 Elm Tree Road
Teddington
Middlesex TW11 8ST
Tel: 020 8977 5474

National Osteoporosis Society
Camerton
Bath BA2 0PJ
Tel: 01761 472721

National Rheumatoid Arthritis
Society
Briarwood House
11 College Avenue
Maidenhead
Berkshire SL6 6AR
Tel: 01628 670606

The Pain Society
21 Portland Place
London W1B 1PY
Tel: 020 7631 8870

Royal College of Nursing
20 Cavendish Square
London W1M 0AB
Tel: 020 7409 3333

Samaritans
Upper Mill
Kingston Road
Ewell
Surrey K17 2AS
Tel: 020 8394 8300

Appendix 4

Guidelines for nurses on the use and administration of intra-articular injections

(By kind permission of the RCN Rheumatology Nursing Forum)

The author has modified these guidelines, as the definitions of extended role and accountability have been discussed within the main text of Chapter 9.

- What are intra-articular injections?

These are injections into the synovial joints. Long-acting steroids are generally used for joint injections and hydrocortisone is used for soft tissue injections.

- Indications for joint injections:
  - (a) Relief of pain from localized inflammation of the joint (e.g. rheumatoid arthritis)
  - (b) Relief of pain from soft tissue discomfort
  - (c) To aid mobilization
  - (d) To assist with rehabilitation (e.g. physiotherapy)
  - (e) To improve function.

- Contraindications for joint injections:
  - (a) Infection
  - (b) Intra-articular fracture
  - (c) Anticoagulant therapy
  - (d) Bleeding disorders.

Preparation the nurse must undertake prior to the administration of intra-articular injections

The nurse must be able to demonstrate evidence of competency in the administration of intra-articular injections in accordance with *The Scope of Professional Practice* (UKCC, 1992). Evidence of competency should indicate that the nurse has knowledge of:

(a) anatomy and physiology of the joints and soft tissues
(b) drugs used and their effects and side effects
(c) indications and contraindications for intra-articular injections
(d) potential complications
(e) aspiration and injection technique.

Evidence of assessment of competency should be available. The employer must have precise knowledge of the employee's activities and agree to them being undertaken by the employee: in accordance with vicarious liability.

- The nurse's responsibility when giving intra-articular injections:
  (a) Obtain written information from the prescribing doctor detailing the drug, dosage and site of administration (Note this practice has been replaced in many units by patient group directions, which will in turn be replaced by the introduction of supplementary prescribing for chronic diseases; DoH, 2003a)
  (b) Ensure that the patient has given informed consent
  (c) Use an aseptic or non-touch technique
  (d) Aspirate the joint if swollen
  (e) Send a sample of synovial fluid for culture if it is very opaque, green or foul smelling
  (f) If no obvious signs of infection or contraindications are present, administer the prescribed drug into the site stated
  (g) Document the drug, dosage and site of administration in the care records.
  (h) Provide the patients with after-care advice.

- After-care advice – the nurse must advise patients that:
  (a) the joint may be painful for 24 hours after the injection. Take analgesia if necessary
  (b) it may take several days before benefit is felt
  (c) the injected joint should be rested for 24-48 hours after the injection
  (d) short-term facial flushing may be experienced
  (e) localized skin atrophy may occasionally occur.

- Potential complications following the administration of intra-articular injections:
  (a) Infections
  (b) Damage to the articular cartilage
  (c) Tendon rupture
  (d) Skin atrophy.

arc leaflet: *Drugs for arthritis – local steroid injections*
2002 version

(Reproduced with the permission of the Arthritis Research Campaign (arc))

Drugs for arthritis - local steroid injections

If you have an inflamed or swollen joint, or if you have pain or inflammation near a joint, your doctor may inject a steroid preparation into the affected area. It is known as a local injection because it acts only in that area. Injecting a joint is called an 'intra- articular' injection. Injecting near a joint but not actually into it is called a 'periarticular' injection (meaning 'near the joint') or 'soft tissue' injection. Sometimes your doctor will inject a local anaesthetic as well as the steroid.

Why do I need a local steroid injection?

An intra-articular injection is given to reduce inflammation, swelling and pain within a joint. A periarticular injection is given to reduce pain and inflammation near a joint. For example, if you have a tennis elbow your doctor may inject the tender area.

How quickly will the steroid injection take to work, and how long will it last?

This varies between different people, but usually improvement starts in one to two days. If it is helpful, the benefit usually lasts from a few weeks to several months.

Are there any side effects?

Side effects are very unlikely. Very occasionally people notice a flare in their joint pain within the first 24 hours after an injection. This usually settles spontaneously over the next couple of days. Very rarely infection might be introduced into the joint at the time of an injection and so if the joint becomes more painful and hot then you should consult your doctor immediately.

Occasionally with periarticular injections some thinning or loss of colour of the skin may occur at the injection site. Local steroid injections may sometimes interfere with the menstrual cycle.

Do I need to rest after the injection?

It is advisable to rest the injected limb as much as possible for the first one to two days after an intra-articular injection.

Where can I obtain further information?

If you would like any further information about steroid injections, or if you have any concerns about your treatment, you should discuss this with your doctor or nurse.

Remember to keep all medicines out of reach of children.

PLEASE NOTE this information sheet does not list all the side effects this drug can cause. For the full details, please see the drug information leaflet that comes with your medicine. Your doctor will assess your medical circumstances and draw your attention to side effects that may be relevant in your particular case.

There are two national organizations in the UK working on behalf of people with arthritis: the Arthritis Research Campaign (address shown below) and Arthritis Care (at 18 Stephenson Way, London NW1 2HD, Tel. 020 7380 6555). Both have agreed the content of this information sheet. For details of other **arc** drugs sheets, please write to the address below, or see our website: www.arc.org.uk.

6250/D-SI/02-1
PUBLISHED BY THE ARTHRITIS RESEARCH CAMPAIGN (arc), COPEMAN HOUSE, ST MARY'S COURT, ST MARY'S GATE, CHESTERFIELD, DERBYSHIRE S41 7TD. REGISTERED CHARITY NO. 207711.

References

Abu-Shakra M, Buskila D, Ehrenfeld M, Conrad K, Shoenfeld Y (2001) Cancer and autoimmunity: autoimmune and rheumatic features in patients with malignancies. Annals of Rheumatic Diseases 60: 433-441.

Adair J (1982) Action Centred Leadership. London: Gower.

Affleck G, Fifield J, Pfieffer C, Tennen H (1998) Social support and psychological adjustment to rheumatoid arthritis. Arthritis Care Research 1: 71-77.

Aletaha D, Smolen JS (2002) Laboratory testing in rheumatoid arthritis patients taking disease modifying anti-rheumatic drugs; clinical evaluation and cost analysis. Arthritis and Rheumatism: Arthritis Care and Research 47: 181-188.

American College of Rheumatology Ad Hoc Committee on Clinical Guidelines (1996) Guidelines for monitoring drug therapy in rheumatoid arthritis. Arthritis and Rheumatism 39: 723-731.

Amgen (2002) Summary of Product Characteristics: anakinra (accessed online at www.emc.vhn.net).

Amgen (2002) Human Interleukin-1 Receptor Antagonist: product monograph. Cambridge: Amgen.

Anttinen J, Oka M (1975) Intra-articular triamcinolone hexacetonide and osmic acid in persistent synovitis of the knee. Scandinavian Journal of Rheumatology 4: 125-128.

Armstrong M (1994) How to be an Effective Manager. London: Kogan Page.

Arnett FC, Edworthy SM, Blotch DA (1988) American Rheumatism Association 1987 revised criteria for the classification of rheumatoid arthritis. Arthritis and Rheumatism 31: 315-324 (www.rheumatology.org).

Arthur V (1994) Nursing care of patients with rheumatoid arthritis. British Journal of Nursing 3: 325-331.

Arthur V (1998) The role of the specialist nurse in rheumatology. In: Le Gallez P (ed). Rheumatology for Nurses: patient care. London: Whurr, pp. 12-45.

Ashcroft J (1999) Understanding People's Everyday Needs. Arthritis - getting it right. A guide for planners. London: Arthritis Care.

Audit Commission (1993) What Seems To Be the Matter? Communication between hospitals and patients. London: HMSO.

Balch HW, Gibson JNC, El-Ghoberey AF, Bain LS, Lynch MP (1997) Repeated corticosteroid injections into lame joints. Rheumatology Rehabilition 16: 137-140.

Bamji AM, Dieppe PA, Haslock DI, Shipley ME (1990) What do rheumatologists do? A pilot audit study. British Journal of Rheumatology 29: 295-298.

Bandolier (2001) Mindstretcher - ranking chronic diseases. January: 83-87.

Bandolier (2002) Adverse drug reactions in hospital patients. (accessed online at www.ebandolier.com).

Bandura A (1977) Self-efficacy; towards a unifying theory of behavioural change. Psychological Review 84: 191-215.

Barry M, Jenner JR (1995) Pain in the neck, shoulder and arm. ABC of Rheumatology. British Medical Journal 310: 183-186.

Beech M (2002) Leaders or managers: the drive for effective leadership. Nursing Standard 16(30): 35-36.

Bellamy N (1993) Musculoskeletal Clinical Metrology. Lancaster: Kluwer Academic Publishers.

Bellamy N, Buchanan WW, Goldsmith CH, Campbell J, Stitt LW (1988) Validation study of WOMAC: a health status instrument for measuring clinically important patient relevant outcomes to antirheumatic drug therapy in patients with osteoarthritis of the hip or knee. Journal of Rheumatology 15: 1833-1840.

Berger RC, Yoint WJ (1990) Immediate steroid flare from intra-articular triamcinolone hexacetonide injection: case report and review of the literature. Arthritis and Rheumatism 33: 1284-1286.

Bird H (1998) Intra-articular and intralesional therapy. In: Klippel JH, Dieppe PA (eds) Rheumatology, 2nd edn. St Louis, MO: Mosby.

Bird HA (1983) Divided rheumatology care; the advent of the nurse practitioner? Annals of Rheumatic Diseases 42: 354-355.

Bird HA, Wright V, Galloway D (1980) Clinical metrology – a future career grade? Lancet ii: 138-140.

Bird HA, Leatham P, Le Gallez P (1981) Clinical metrology. Nursing Times 77: 1926-1927.

Blaxter M (1992) Health and Lifestyles. London: Tavistock Routledge.

Blyth T, Hunter JA, Stirling A (1994) Pain relief in the rheumatoid knee after steroid injection: a single blind comparison of hydrocortisone succinate and triamcinolone acetonide or hexacetonide. British Journal of Rheumatology 33: 461-463.

Bowling A (1997) Measuring Health: a review of quality of life measurement scales, 2nd edn. Buckingham: Open University Press.

Bowling A (2001) Measuring Disease: a review of disease-specific quality of life measurement scales, 2nd edn. Buckingham: Open University Press.

Braun J, Sieper J, Breban M, Collantes-Estevez E, Davis J, Inman R, Marzo-Ortega H, Mielants H (2002) Anti-tumour necrosis factor alpha therapy for ankylosing spondylitis: international experience. Annals of Rheumatic Diseases 61(Supplement iii): 51-60.

Bresnihan B (2000) Product Monograph. Cambridge: Amgen.

Bresnihan B (2001) The safety and efficacy of interleukin-1 receptor antagonist in the treatment of rheumatoid arthritis. Seminars in Arthritis and Rheumatism 30(Supplement II): 17-20.

Bresnihan B (2002) Effects on anakinra on clinical and radiological outcomes in rheumatoid arthritis. Annals of Rheumatic Diseases 61(Supplement ii): ii74-ii77.

Bresnihan B, Alvaro-Gracia JM, Cobby M et al. (1998) Treatment of rheumatoid arthritis with recombinant human interleukin-1 receptor antagonist. Arthritis and Rheumatism 41: 2196-2204.

British League Against Rheumatism (1997) Arthritis Getting it Right: a guide for planners. London: British League Against Rheumatism.

British Paediatric Rheumatology Group (2000) Guidelines for Prescribing Biologic Therapies in Children and Young People with Juvenile Idiopathic Arthritis. London: British Paediatric Rheumatology Group.

British Society for Rheumatology (1992) Report of a Joint Working Group of the British Society for Rheumatology and the Royal College of Physicians of London. Guidelines and audit measures for the specialist supervision of patients with rheumatoid arthritis, Journal of Royal College of Physicians, London 26: 76-82.

British Society for Rheumatology (1994) Musculoskeletal Disorders: providing for the patient's needs. London: British Society for Rheumatology.

British Society for Rheumatology (2000) Guidelines for Second Line Drug Monitoring. London: British Society for Rheumatology.

British Society for Rheumatology (2002) Providing for the Patient's Needs. The role of the rheumatology department, epidemiological based estimates of manpower requirements, and a basis for planning a rheumatology service. London: British Society for Rheumatology.

British Society for Rheumatology (2003) Guidelines for Prescribing Tumour Necrosis Factor Alpha Blockers in Adults with Rheumatoid Arthritis. London: British Society for Rheumatology.

British Society for Rheumatology Working Party (2000) New Treatments in Rheumatoid Arthritis: the use of TNFa blockers in adults with rheumatoid arthritis. London: British Society for Rheumatology, pp. 1–9.

Broadcastive Support Services Telephone Helpline Groups (1993) Telephone Helplines; guidelines for good practice, 2nd edn. London: Windsor Print Production.

Brocklehurst N, Clark J, Clegg A (1999) Getting into business: how nurses can make a difference. Nursing Standard 14(2): 46–53.

Brocklehurst N, Walshe K (1999) Quality and the new NHS. Nursing Standard 13(51): 46–53.

Brownsell C, Dawson JK (2002) Rheumatology telephone helpline services. Rheumatology 41: 710–711.

Bury M (1988) Chronic illness as a biographical disruption. Sociology of Health and Illness 4: 167–182.

Butterworth T (1997) It is Good to Talk. An evaluation study of clinical supervision in 23 sites in England and Scotland. Manchester: University of Manchester School of Nursing, Midwifery and Health Visiting.

Byrne J (1998) Medication in rheumatic disease. In: Hill J (ed.) Rheumatology Nursing: a creative approach. Edinburgh: Churchill Livingstone.

Caine N, Sharples LD, Hollingworth W et al. (2002) A randomised controlled crossover trial of nurse practitioner versus doctor-led outpatient care in a bronchiectasis clinic. Health Technology Assessment. NHS Research and Development HTA Programme 6(27). Southampton: The National Co-ordinating Centre for Health technology Assessment.

Callahan LF, Bloch DA, Pincus T (1992) Identification of work disability in rheumatoid arthritis: physical, radiographic and laboratory variable do not add explanatory power to demographic and functional variables. Journal of Clinical Epidemiology 45: 127–138.

Cameron C (1996) Patient compliance: recognition of factors involved and suggestions for promoting compliance with therapeutic regimens. Journal of Advanced Nursing 24: 244–250.

Cameron G (1995) Steroid arthropathy: myth or reality? Journal of Orthopaedic Medicine 17(2): 51–55.

Canoso JJ (1998) Aspiration and injection of joints and periarticular tissues. In: Klippel JH, Dieppe PA (eds) Rheumatology, 2nd edn. St Louis, MO: Mosby.

Cappell HA, Hampsom R, McCarey D, Madhok R (2001) '5D' assessment in a 20 year follow up of 123 rheumatoid arthritis patients. Arthritis and Rheumatism 9(44): S220.

Carr AJ (1996) A patient centered approach to the evaluation and treatment in RA: the development of a clinical tool to measure patient perceived handicap. British Journal of Rheumatology 35: 921–932.

Carr AJ (2001) Defining the extended clinical role for allied health professionals in rheumatology. Conference Proceedings 12. Chesterfield: Arthritis Research Campaign.

Carter S, Taylor D, Levenson R (2003) A Question of Choice – Compliance in Medicine Taking: a preliminary review. London: Medicines Partnership.

Casey ATH, Crockard A (1995) Topics in Orthopaedic Surgery: In the rheumatoid patient: surgery to the cervical spine. British Journal of Rheumatology 34: 1078–1086.

Castledine G (1994) Specialist and advanced nursing and the scope of practice. In: Hunt G, Wainwright P (eds) Expanding the Role of the Nurse; the scope of professional practice. Oxford: Blackwell Science, pp. 101–112.

Castledine G (1999) Developments in the role of the advanced nursing practitioner: a personal perspective. In: Rolfe G, Fulbrook P (eds) Advanced Nursing Practice. Oxford: Butterworth-Heinemann.

Cawley PJ, Morris IM (1992) A study to compare the efficacy of two methods of skin preparation for joint injections. British Journal of Rheumatology 31: 847-848.

Chakravarty K, Pharoah PDP, Scott DGI (1994) A randomised controlled study of post-injection rest following intra-articular steroid therapy for knee synovitis. British Journal of Rheumatology 33: 464-468.

Challinor P (1999) Meetings: the challenge. Nursing Standard 13(50): 40-45.

Chambers N, Jolly A (2002) Essence of care; making a difference. Nursing Standard 17(11): 40-44.

Charmaz K (1983) Loss of self: a fundamental form of suffering in the chronically ill. Sociology of Health and Ilness 5: 168-195.

Cheifetz A, Mayer L, Plevy S (2001) The incidence and management of infusion reactions to infliximab: a large centre experience. Abstract presented at the American College of Gastroenterology 66th Annual Scientfic Meeting, Las Vegas, October.

Choy EHS, Panayi G (2001) Cytokine pathways and joint inflammation in rheumatoid arthritis. New England Journal of Medicine 344: 907-915.

Claus K, Bailey J (1997) Power and Conference in Healthcare. A new approach to leadership. St Louis, MO: Mosby.

Coleman A (1997) Where do I stand? Legal implications of telephone triage. Journal of Clinical Nursing 6: 227-231.

Comer M, Scott DL, Doyle DV, Huskisson EC, Hopkins A (1995) Are slow acting anti-rheumatic drugs monitored too often? An audit of current clinical practice. British Journal of Rheumatology 34: 966-970.

Commission for Health Improvement (2002) Discussion Paper. Guidelines for the NHS on establishing and running help lines. London: Commission for Health Improvement.

Comptroller and Auditor General (2002) NHS Direct in England. London: The Stationery Office.

Cooper C, Kirwan JR (1990) The risk of local and systemic corticosteroid administration. Baillière's Clinical Rheumatology. London: Baillière Tindall.

Coote A, Appleby J (2002) Five Year Health Check. A review of government health policy 1997-2002. London: King's Fund.

Corbin JM, Strauss A (1988) Unending Work and Care. San Francisco, CA: Jossey Bass.

Corcoran M (1999) The Legal Aspects of Prescribing and Monitoring. Presentation at 'Bridging the Gap' Conference, North Devon, April 1999.

Cornell P, Trehance A, Benjamin S, Thick G, Taylor J, Thompson P, Hunt R (1999) Telephone helpline audit. Rheumatology 38(Supplement 1): 170.

Creed F (1990) Psychological disorders in rheumatoid arthritis; a growing consensus? Annals of Rheumatic Diseases 49: 808-812.

Crosby LJ (1991) Factors which contribute to fatigue associated with rheumatoid arthritis. Journal of Advanced Nursing 16: 974-981.

Crouch R, Dale J (1998) Telephone triage - identifying the demand. Nursing Standard 12: 33-38.

Crouch R, Woodfield H, Dale J, Patel A (1997) Telepone assessment and advice; a training programme. Nursing Standard 11(47): 41-44.

Davis RM, Wagner G, Groves T (2002) Advances in managing chronic disease. Research, performance measurement, and quality improvement are key. British Medical Journal 320: 525-526.

De Jong Z, Van Der Heijde D, McKenna SP, Whalley D (1997) The reliability and construct validity of the RAQoL: a rheumatoid arthritis-specific quality of life instrument. British Journal of Rheumatology: 36: 878-883.

De Luc K (2001) Developing Care Pathways: the handbook. Oxford: Radcliffe Medical Press.

De Wolf AN, Mens JMA (1994) Can corticosteroid cause menstrual bleeding? Vademecum 12: 7.

den Broeder AA, Creemers MCW, van Gestel AM, Van Riel PLCM (2002) Dose titration using the Disease Activity Score (DAS 28) in rheumatoid arthritis patients treated with anti-TNFa. Rheumatology 41: 638–642.

Department of Health (1989) The Patient's Charter: working for patients. London: Department of Health.

Department of Health (1996) Promoting Clinical Effectiveness: a framework for action in and through the NHS. London: Department of Health.

Department of Health (1997) The New NHS: modern, dependable. London: Department of Health.

Department of Health (1998) A First Class Service. London: Department of Health.

Department of Health (1999a) Making a Difference. Strengthening the nursing and health visiting contribution to health and healthcare. London: Department of Health.

Department of Health (1999b) Quality and Performance in the NHS: performance assessment framework. London: Department of Health.

Department of Health (1999c) Clinical Governance: quality in the new NHS. London: Department of Health.

Department of Health (1999d) Making a Difference. Reducing burdens in hospitals. Public sector impact unit. London: Department of Health.

Department of Health (2000a) The NHS Plan. London: Department of Health.

Department of Health (2000b) A Plan for Investment, a Plan for Reform. London: Department of Health.

Department of Health (2001a) Shifting the Balance of Power: securing delivery. London: Department of Health.

Department of Health (2001b) The Expert Patient: a new approach to chronic disease management for the 21st century. London: Department of Health.

Department of Health (2001c) The Essence of Care. London: Department of Health.

Department of Health (2001d) Good Practice in Consent: implementation guide. London: Department of Health.

Department of Health (2001e) Reference Guide to Consent for Examination and Treatment. London: Department of Health.

Department of Health (2001f) Health and Social Care Act. London: Department of Health.

Department of Health (2002a) NHS Modernisation Agenda: clinical governance. London: Department of Health.

Department of Health (2002b) Shifting the Balance of Power: the next steps. London: Department of Health.

Department of Health (2002c) NHS Reform and Healthcare Professions Act. London: Department of Health.

Department of Health (2003a) Supplementary Prescribing by Nurses and Pharmacists within the NHS in England. A guide for implementation. London: Department of Health.

Department of Health (2003b) Strengthening Accountability: involving patients and the public. London: Department of Health.

Department of Health (2003c) Modern Matrons – improving the patient experience. London: Department of Health.

Department of Health (2003d) Agenda for Change: proposed agreement. London: Department of Health.

Devlin R (1999) The Write Stuff. Nursing Standard 95(48): 26–28.

Dieppe PA, Sathapatyavongs B, Jones HE et al. (1980) Intra-articular steroids in osteoarthritis. Rheumatology and Rehabilitation 19: 212–217.

Dimond B (1994) Legal aspects of role expansion. In: Hunt G, Wainwright P (eds) Expanding the Role of the Nurse: the scope of professional practice. Oxford: Blackwell Science.

Dimond B (2002) Legal Aspects of Nursing. Harlow: Prentice Hall.

Dinarello CA, Moldawer LL (2000) Pro-inflammatory and Anti-inflammatory Cytokines in Rheumatoid Arthritis. California: Amgen.

Doherty M, Hazelman B, Hutton CW et al. (1992) Rheumatology Examination and Injection Techniques. London: WB Saunders, pp. 123-127.

Dorman T, Ravin T (1991) Diagnosis and Injection Techniques in Orthopaedic Medicine. Baltimore, MD: Williams & Wilkins, pp. 33-34.

Dowling S, Martyn R, Skidmore P et al. (1996) Nurses taking on junior doctors work: a confusion of accountability. British Medical Journal 312: 1211-1214.

Edwards J, Hannah B, Brailsford-Atkinson K, Price T, Sheeran T, Mulherin D (2002) Intra-articular and soft tissue injections: assessment of the service provided by nurses. Annals of Rheumatic Disease 61: 6656-6657.

Edwards J, Hassell A (2000) Intra-articular and soft tissue injections by nurses: preparation for expanded practice. Nursing Standard 14(33): 43.

Egleston C, Kelly H, Cope A (1994) Use of a telephone advice line in accident and emergency. British Medical Journal 308: 31.

Elliott K (2001) Implementing nursing clinical indicators. Professional Nurse 16: 1158-1161.

Embrey N, Lowndes C, Warner R (2003) Benchmarking best practice in relapse management of multiple sclerosis. Nursing Standard 17(22): 38-42.

Emery P, Salmon M (1995) Early rheumatoid arthritis; time to aim for remission. Annals of Rheumatic Disease 54: 944-947.

Emery P, Panayi G, Sturrock R, Williams B (1999) Targeted therapies in rheumatoid arthritis: the need for action. Rheumatology 38: 911-916.

Emery P, Breedveld FC, Dougados M, Kalden JR, Schiff MH, Smolen JS (2002) Early referral recommendations for newly diagnosed rheumatoid arthritis; evidence based developments of a clinical guide. Annals of Rheumatic Diseases 61: 290-297.

Emkey RD, Lindsay R, Lyssy J, Weisberg J, Dempster DW, Shen V (1996) The systemic effects of intra-articular administration of corticosteroid markers of bone formation and bone resorption in patients with rheumatoid arthritis. Arthritis Rheumatism 39: 277-282.

Felson DT, Anderson JJ, Boers M (1993) The American College of Rheumatology preliminary core set of disease activity measures for rheumatoid arthritis clinical trials. The committee on outcome measures in rheumatoid arthritis clinical trials. Arthritis and Rheumatism 36: 729-740.

Fransen J, Stucki G, van Riel P (2002) The merits of monitoring; should we follow all our rheumatoid arthritis patients in daily practice? Rheumatology 41: 601-604.

Fries JF, Spitz P, Kraines RG, Holman HR (1980) Measurement of patient outcome in arthritis: Arthritis and Rheumatism 23: 137-145.

Fries JF (2000) Current treatment paradigms in rheumatoid arthritis. Rheumatology 39(Supplement 1): 30-35.

Fuchs HA, Brooks RH, Callahan LF, Pincus T (1989) A simplified twenty-eight joint quantitative articular index in rheumatoid arthritis. Arthritis and Rheumatism 32: 531-537.

Furst DE, Breedveld FC, Kalden JR et al. (2002) Updated consensus statement on biological agents for the treatment of rheumatoid arthritis and other rheumatic diseases. Annals of Rheumatic Diseases 61(Supplement ii): 2-7.

Gaffney K, Ledingham J, Perry JD et al. (1995) Intra-articular triamcinolone hexacetonide in knee osteoarthritis: factors influencing the clinical response. Annals of Rheumatic Disease 54: 379-381.

George S (2002) NHS Direct audited; customer satisfaction what price? British Medical Journal 324: 558-559.

Gerhardht U (1990) Qualitative research on chronic illness: the issue and the story. Social Science and Medicine 30: 1149-1159.

Gray RG, Tenenbaum J, Gottlieb NL (1981) Local corticosteroid injection therapy in rheumatic orders. Seminars in Arthritis and Rheumatism 10: 231-254.

Grimshaw J, Freemantle N, Wallace S et al. (1995) Developing and implementing clinical practice guidelines. Quality in Health Care 4: 55-64.

Grove ML, Hassell AB, Hay EM, Shadforth MF (2001)Adverse reactions to disease modifying anti-rheumatic drugs in clinical practice. Quarterly Journal of Medicine 94: 309-319.

Guest D, Redfern S, Wilson-Barnett J et al. (2001) A Preliminary Evaluation of the Establishment of Nurse, Midwife and Health Visitor Consultants. London: King's College London.

Hallam I (1989) You've got a lot to answer for Mr. Bell. A review of the use of the telephone in primary care. Family Practice 6: 47-57.

Haslock I, MacFarlane D, Speed C (1995) Intra-articular and soft tissue injections: a survey of current practice. British Journal of Rheumatology 34: 449-452.

Havelock M (1998) Audit of compliance of slow acting anti-rheumatic and cytotoxic agents in rheumatology outpatients. Conference presentation, Royal College of Nursing Rheumatology Forum, Bath.

Hawley DJ (1995) Psycho-education interventions for the treatment of arthritis. Clinical Rheumatology 9: 803-823.

Hawley DJ, Wolfe F (1998) Anxiety and depression in patients with rheumatoid arthritis: a prospective study of 400 patients. Journal Rheumatology 5: 932-941.

Hay EM, Bacon PA, Gorden C, Isenberg DA et al. (1993) The BILAG index: a reliable and valid instrument for measuring clinical disease activity in systemic lupus erythematosus. Quarterly Journal of Medicine 86: 447-458.

Haynes J, Dieppe P (1993) Increasing awareness of arthritis - the public's response. British Journal of Rheumatology 32: 623-624.

Hazes JMW, Hayton R, Burt J, Silman AJ (1994) Consistency of morning stiffness; an analysis of diary data. British Journal of Rheumatology 33: 562-565.

Helliwell PS, O'Hara M (1995) Shared DMARD monitoring. British Journal of Rheumatology 36: 926-927.

Hewlett S, Cockshott ZC, Kirwan JR, Barrett J, Stamp J, Haslock I (2001a) Development and validation of a self-efficacy scale for use in British patients with rheumatoid arthritis (RASE). Rheumatology 40: 1221-1230.

Hewlett S, Mitchell K, Hayes J (2001b) A shared care system of hospital follow up reduced pain and use of healthcare resources and increase satisfaction inpatients with rheumatoid arthritis. Evidence Based Nursing 4: 51.

Hewlett S, Smith AP, Kirwan JR (2002) Measuring the meaning of disability in rheumatoid arthritis: the Personal Impact Health Assessment Questionnaire (PI HAQ). Annals of Rheumatic Disease 61: 986-993.

Hill J (1985) Nursing clinics for arthritics. Nursing Times 18: 33-34.

Hill J (1986) Patient evaluation of rheumatology nursing clinics. Nursing Times 82: 42-43.

Hill J (1995) Patient education in rheumatic diseases. Nursing Standard 9: 25-28.

Hill J (1997) Patient satisfaction in a nurse led rheumatology clinic. Journal of Advanced Nursing 25: 347-354.

Hill J (1998a) Rheumatology Nursing: a creative approach. Edinburgh: Churchill Livingstone.

Hill J (1998b) Pain and stiffness. In: Hill J (ed.) Rheumatology Nursing: a creative approach. Edinburgh: Churchill Livingstone, pp. 137-153.

Hill J (1999) Patient education and adherence to drug therapy. In: Hill J, Ryan S. Drug Therapy in Rheumatology Nursing. London: Whurr, pp. 211-258.

Hill J (2003) An overview of patient education in the rheumatic diseases. Nursing Times (in press).

Hill J, Bird HA, Harmer R, Wright V, Lawton C (1994) An evaluation of the effectiveness, safety and acceptability of a nurse practitioner in a rheumatology outpatient clinic. British Journal of Rheumatology 33: 282-288.

Hill J, Bird H, Johnson S (2001) Effect of patient education on adherence to drug treatment for rheumatoid arthritis; a randomised controlled trial. Annals of Rheumatic Diseases 60: 869-875.

Hill J, Thorpe R, Bird H (2003a) Outcomes for patients with RA - a rheumatology nurse practitioner clinic compared to standard outpatient care. Musculoskeletal Care 1(1): 5-20.

Hill J, Bird H, Thorpe R (2003b) Effects of rheumatoid arthritis on sexual activity and relationships. Rheumatology 42: 280-286.

Hirano PC, Laurent DD, Lorig K (1994) Arthritis patient education studies. 1987-1991 a review of the literature. Patient Education and Counselling 24: 9-54.

Hoffbrand AV, Pettit JE (1993) Essential Haematology, 3rd edn. Oxford: Blackwell Scientific Publications.

Hollander JL (1970) Intrasynovial corticosteroid therapy in arthritis. Medical State Medicine Journal 19: 62-66.

Hollander JL, Brown EM IR, Jessar RA, Brown CY (1951) Hydrocortisone and cortisone injected into arthritic joints: comparative effects of the use of hydrocortisone as a local anaesthetic agent. Journal of the American Medical Association 147: 1629-1635.

Holman H and Lorig K (2000) Patients as partners in managing chronic disease. British Medical Journal 320: 526-527.

Hommes D (2003) Inflammatory bowel disease. Presentation at 1st International Conference on Cytokine Medicine, Manchester, February.

Horrocks S, Anderson E, Salisbury C (2002) Systematic review of whether nurse practitioners working in primary care can provide equivalent care to doctors. British Medical Journal 324: 819-823.

Hughes RA (2003) Telephone helplines in rheumatology. Rheumatology 42: 197-9.

Hughes RA, Carr ME, Huggett A, Thwaites CEA (2002) Review of the function of a telephone helpline in the treatment of outpatients with rheumatoid arthritis. Annals of Rheumatic Diseases 61: 341-345.

Humphris D (ed.) (1994) The Clinical Nurse Specialist: issues in practice. London: Macmillan.

Hunt C, Stark JL, Fisher F, Hegedus K, Joy L, Woldum K (1983) Networking a managerial strategy for research development in a service setting. Journal of Nursing Administration 13: 31-32.

Hunt G (1994) New professionals? New ethics? In: Hunt G, Wainwright P (eds) Expanding the Role of the Nurse. Oxford: Blackwell.

Hunt G, Evans W (1994) Health care assistants and accountability. In: Hunt G, Wainwright P (eds) Expanding the Role of the Nurse. Oxford: Blackwell.

Hunt G, Wainwright P (eds) (1994) Expanding the Role of the Nurse. Oxford: Blackwell.

Huskisson E (1982) Measurement of pain. Journal of Rheumatology 9: 768-769.

Iles V, Sutherland K (2001) Organisational Change – managing change in the NHS. London: National Co-ordinating Centre/Service Development Organisation.

International Liaison Committee on Resuscitation (ILCOR) (1997) Special resuscitation situations. Resuscitation 34: 140-141.

Isenberg D, Morrow J (1995) Friendly Fire: explaining auto-immune disease. Oxford: Oxford University Press.

Jacobs LG, Barton MA, Wallace WA, Ferrousis J, Dunn NA, Bossingham DA (1991) Intra-articular distension and corticosteroids in the management of capsulitis of the shoulder. British Medical Journal 302: 1498-1501.

Janowski J (1995) Is telephone triage calling you? American Journal of Nursing 95: 59-62.

Jeyasingham M (1999) Higher level practice: the consumer's perspective. Professional Nurse 14: 311-314.

Jiang Y, Genant HK, Watt I et al. (2000) A multicenter, double blind, dose ranging randomised placebo controlled study of recombinant human interleukin-1 receptor antagonist in patients with rheumatoid arthritis. Arthritis and Rheumatism 43: 1001-1009.

Joint Tuberculosis Committee of the British Thoracic Society (2003) Recommendations for assessing risk and for managing M. tuberculosis infection and disease in patients due to start anti-TNF alpha treatment. Presentation at 1st International Conference on Cytokine Medicine, Manchester, February.

Jones A, Doherty M (1996) Intra-articular corticosteroids are effective in osteoarthritis but there are no clinical predictors of response. Annals of Rheumatic Disease 55: 829–832.

Jones A, Regan M, Ledingham J, Pattrick M, Manhire A, Doherty M (1993) Importance of placement of intra-articular steroid injections. British Medical Journal 307: 1329–1330.

Kaufmann SHE (2002) Protection against tuberculosis; cytokines, T cells and macrophages. Annals of Rheumatic Diseases 61 Supp ii: 54–58.

Kay E (1991) Methylprednislone acetate: a pharmacological review. In: Focus on Depromedrone. London: Haywood Medical Communications, pp. 6–11.

Kay EA, Pullar T (1993) Variation among rheumatologists in prescribing and monitoring anti-rheumatic drugs. British Journal of Rheumatology 31: 477–483.

Keane J, Gershon S, Pharm D et al. (2001) Tuberculosis associated with infliximab, a tumour necrosis factor a-neutralizing agent. New England Journal of Medicine 345: 1098–1104.

Keystone EC (2003) Advances in targeted therapy: safety of biological agents. Annals of Rheumatic Diseases 62 Supp ii: 34–36

Kiely PDW, Johnson DM (2002) Infliximab and leflunomide combination therapy in rheumatoid arthritis: an open label study. Rheumatology 41: 631–637.

Kirkham B (2003) Infliximab treatment of psoriatic arthritis. Presentation at 1st International Conference on Cytokine Medicine, Manchester, February.

Kirwan J (1997) Rheumatology outpatient workload increases inexorably. Journal of Rheumatology 36: 481–486.

Kirwan J, Haskard DO, Higgens CS (1984) The use of sequential analysis to assess patient preference for local skin anaesthetic during knee aspiration. British Journal of Rheumatology 23: 210–213.

Kirwan JR, Reeback JS (1986) Standford Health Assessment Questionnaire modified to assess disability in British patients with rheumatoid arthritis. British Journal of Rheumatology 25: 206–209.

Kitson A (1993) Setting up a network. Nursing Standard 7(27): 7–8.

Kleinman A (1988) The Illness Narrative: suffering, healing and the human condition. New York: Harper Collins.

Labelle H, Guilbert R, Joncas, J, Newman, N, Fallaha M, Richard CH (1992) Lack of scientific evidence for the treatment of lateral epicondylitis of the elbow. Journal of Bone and Joint Surgery 74B: 646–651.

Lattimer V, Sassi F, George S, Moore M, Turnbull J, Mullee M (2002) Cost analysis of nurse telephone consultation in out of hours primary care; evidence from a randomised controlled trial. British Medical Journal 324: 1053–1057.

Le Gallez P (1993) Rheumatoid arthritis; effects on the family. Nursing Standard 7: 30–34.

Le Gallez P (ed.) (1998) Rheumatology for Nurses: patient care. London: Whurr.

Lewis CE, Resnik BA (1967) Nurse clinics and progressive ambulatory patient care. New England Journal of Medicine 277: 1236–1241.

Lewis CE, Resnik BA, Schmidt G, Waxman D (1969) Activities, events and outcomes in ambulatory patient care. New England Journal of Medicine 280: 645–649.

Lipsky PE, ven der Heijde DM, St Clair EW et al. (2000) Infliximab and methorexate in the treatment of rheumatoid arthritis. New England Journal of Medicine 22: 1594–1602.

Lorig K (1996) Patient Education – a practical approach. Thousand Oaks, CA: Sage.

Lorig K, Konkol L, Gonzalez V (1987) Arthritis patient education; a review of the literature. Patient Education and Counselling 10: 207–252.

Lorig K, Chastain R, Ung E, Shoor S, Holman H (1989) Development and evaluation of a scale to measure perceived self-efficacy in people with arthritis. Arthritis and Rheumatism 32: 37–44.

Lovell DJ, Giannini EH, Reiff A et al. (2003) Long-term efficacy and safety of etanercept in children with polyarticular-course juvenile rheumatoid arthritis. Arthritis and Rheumatism 48: 218–226.

Mace S, Vadas P, Pruzanski W (1997) Anaphylactic shock induced by intra-articular injection of methylprednisolone acetate. Journal of Rheumatology 24: 1191-1194.

Maddison P (2001) Development of current management strategies. In: Haslock I, Pitzalis C, Reeves B, Shipley M (eds) Key Advances in the Effective Management of Rheumatoid Arthritis. London: Royal Society of Medicine.

Maini RN (2002) Biologic mediators and advanced therapies in rheumatoid arthritis. Presentation at Asia Pacific League Against Rheumatism Conference, Thailand.

Maini RN, Feldman M, Kalden JR et al. (1998) Therapeutic efficacy of multiple intravenous infusions of anti-tumour necrosis factor alpha monoclonal antibody combined with low dose weekly methotrexate in rheumatoid arthritis. Arthritis and Rheumatism 41: 1552-1563.

Marklund B, Koritz P, Bjorkander E, Bengtsson C (1991) How well do nurse-run telephone consultations and consultations in the surgery agree? Experience in Swedish primary health care. British Journal of General Practice 41: 462-465.

McCabe C, McDowell J, Cushnaghan J, Butts S, Hewlett S, Stafford S (2000) Rheumatology telephone helplines: an activity analysis. Rheumatology 39: 1390-1395.

McFarlane AC, Brooks PM (1988) Determinants of disability in rheumatoid arthritis. British Journal of Rheumatology 27: 7-14.

McSherry R, Kell J, Pearce P (2002) Clinical supervision and clinical governance. Nursing Times 98(23): 30-32.

Medicines Control Agency (2002) Extensions of the Yellow Card Scheme to Nurse Reporters; suspected adverse drug reactions reporting. London: Medicines Control Agency.

Meenan RF, Gertman PM, Mason JM (1980) Measuring health status in arthritis; the Arthritis Impact Measurement Scale. Arthritis and Rheumatism 23: 146-153.

Meenan RF, Mason JH, Anderson JJ, Guccione AA, Kazis LE (1992) AIMS 2. The content and properties of a revised and expanded Arthritis Impact Measurement Scales health status questionnaire. Arthritis and Rheumatism 35: 1-10.

Millard RS, Dillingham MF (1995) Peripheral joint injections: lower extremity. Physical Medicine and Rehabilitation Clinics of North America 6: 841-849.

Miller L (2002) Telephone clinic improves quality of follow up care for chronic bowel disease. Nursing Times 98(31): 36-38.

Moldofsky H, Chester WJ (1970) Pain and mood patterns in people with rheumatoid arthritis. Psychosomatic Medicine 32: 309-318.

Mooney J (1999) Bridging the gap between primary and secondary care: Rheumatology Nursing outreach clinics. Poster presentation at EULAR Congress, Glasgow.

Moots R, Taggart A, Walker D (2003) Biologic therapy in clinical practice: enthusiasm must be tempered by caution. Rheumatology 42: 614-615.

Mulherin D, Fitzgerald O, Bresnihan B (1996) Clinical improvement and radiological deterioration in rheumatoid arthritis: evidence that the pathogenesis of synovial inflammation and articular erosion may differ. British Journal of Rheumatology 35: 1263-1268.

National Institute for Clinical Excellence (2001) National Institute for Clinical Excellence (NICE) response to Department of Heatlh announcement on new statutory obligations for NHS to fund treatments recommended by NICE. Press Media Report.

National Institute for Clinical Excellence (2002a) Guidance on the use of Etanercept and Infliximab for the Treatment of Rheumatoid Arthritis. London: NICE.

National Institute for Clinical Excellence (2002b) Principles of Best Practice in Clinical Audit. Oxford: Radcliffe Medical Press.

National Institute for Clinical Excellence (2002c) Etanercept for Juvenile Idiopathic Arthritis. London: NICE.

National Institute for Clinical Excellence (2003a) What is Protocol Based Care? London: NICE.

National Institute for Clinical Excellence (2003b) Technology Assessment Report commissioned by the HTA Programme on behalf of the National Institute for Clinical Excellence: the clinical and cost-effectiveness of anakinra for the treatment of RA in adults. (Accessed online at www.nice.org.uk).

National Patient Safety Agency (2002) Annual Report 2001-2002. London: National Patient Safety Agency.

Neustadt DH (1985) Synovitis of the knee. Effects of a post injection rest. Clinical Rheumatology Practice 3: 65-68.

Neustadt DH (1991) Local corticosteroid injection therapy in soft tissue rheumatic conditions of the hand and wrist. Arthritis and Rheumatism 34: 923-926.

Newbold D (1996) Psychological assessment in rheumatic disease. Journal of Clinical Nursing 5: 373-380.

NHS Executive (1997) The New NHS: modern and dependable. A national framework for assessing performance: consultation document. London: Department of Health.

NHS Modernisation Agency (2001) 27 Key Principles for Service Redesign. London: NHS Executive.

NHS Modernisation Agency and National Institute for Clinical Excellence (2002) Protocol Based Care. Underpinning improvement. London: Department of Health.

NHS Modernisation Agency and Department of Health (2003) Essence of Care: patient-focused benchmarks for clinical governance. London: Department of Health.

Nicassio PM, Wallston KA, Callahan LF, Herbert M, Pincus T (1985) The measurement of helplessness in rheumatoid arthritis: the development of the Arthritis Helplessness Index. Journal of Rheumatology 12: 642-647.

Nicklin J (2002) Improving the quality of written information for patients. Nursing Standard 16(49): 39-44.

Nuki G, Bresnihan B, Bear MB, McCabe D (2002) Long term safety and maintenace of clincal improvement following treatment with anakinra (recombinant human Interleukin-1 receptor antagonist) in patients with rheumatoid arthritis. Arthritis and Rheumatism 46: 2838-2846.

Nursing and Midwifery Council (2002a) Guidelines for records and record keeping. London: Nursing and Midwifery Council.

Nursing and Midwifery Council (2002b) Code of Professional Conduct. London: Nursing and Midwifery Council.

Nursing and Midwifery Council (2002c) Guidelines for the administration of medicines. London: Nursing and Midwifery Council.

Oberai B, Kirwan JR (1988) Psychological factors in patients with chronic rheumatoid arthritis. Annals of Rheumatic Diseases 32: 969-971.

O'Cathain A, Munro JF, Nicholls JP, Knowles E (2000) How helpful is NHS Direct? Postal survey of callers. British Medical Journal 320: 1035.

Oliver S (1997) Rheumatology shared care monitoring audit. Unpublished. Northern Devon Healthcare Trust audit report.

Oliver S (1999) Rheumatology shared care monitoring reaudit. Unpublished. Northern Devon Healthcare Trust re-audit report.

Oliver S, Mooney J (2002) Targeted therapies for patients with rheumatoid arthritis. Professional Nurse 17: 716-780.

Oliver SM (2001) Living with failing lungs; the doctor-patient relationship. Family Practice 18: 430-439.

Owen DS (1997) Aspiration and injection of joints and soft tissues. In: Kelly WN, Harris ED, Ruddy S, Sledge CB (eds) Textbook of Rheumatology, vol. 1, 5th edn. London: WB Saunders, pp. 591-608.

Parker GM (1990) Team Players and Teamwork. The new competitive business strategy. San Francisco, CA: Jossey Bass.

Parker JC, Wright GE (1995) The implications of depression for pain and disability in rheumatoid arthritis. Arthritis Care Research 8: 279-283.

Patel A, Dale J, Crouch R (1997) Satisfaction with telephone advice from an accident and emergency department; identifying areas for service improvement. Quality in Health Care 6: 140-145.

Pennels C (1997) Nursing and the law: clinical responsibility. Professional Nurse 13:162-164.

Phelan MJ, Byrne J, Campbell A, Lynch M (1992) A profile of rheumatology nurse specialist in the United Kingdom. British Journal of Rheumatology 31: 858-859.

Pincus T, Callahan LF (1993) The 'side effects' of rheumatoid arthritis: joint destruction, disability and early mortality. British Journal of Rheumatology 32 Supp 1: 28-37.

Pincus T, Sokka T (2001) Quantitative target values of predictors of mortality in rheumatoid arthritis as possible goals for therapeutic interventions: an alternative approach to remission or ACR 20 response? Journal of Rheumatology 28: 1723-1734.

Pincus T, Summey JA, Soraci SA, Wallston KA, Hummon NP (1983) Assessment of patient satisfaction in activities of daily living using a modified Stanford Health Assessment Questionnaire. Arthritis and Rheumatism 26: 1346-1353.

Pincus T, Marcum S, Callahan L (1992) Long term drug therapy for rheumatoid arthritis in seven rheumatology private practices. Second line drugs and prednisolone. Journal of Rheumatology 19: 1885-1894.

Pincus T, Ferraccioli G, Sokka T et al. (2002) Evidence from clinical trials and long term observational studies that disease-modifying anti-rheumatic drugs slow radiographic progression in rheumatoid arthritis; updating a 1983 review. Rheumatology 41: 1346-1356.

Pirmohamed M, Breckenridge AM, Kitteringham NR, Kevin Park B (1998) Adverse drug reactions. British Medical Journal 316: 1295-1298.

Pisetsky DS (2000) Tumour necrosis factor blockers in rheumatoid arthritis. New England Journal of Medicine 342: 808-811.

Plant M (2001) Diagnosis: clinical, laboratory and imaging. London: Royal Society of Medicine.

Platt S, Tannahill A, Watson J, Fraser E. (1997) Effectiveness of anti-smoking telephone helpline: follow up survey. British Medical Journal 314: 1371-1375.

Polgar S, Thomas S (1998) Introduction to Research in the Health Sciences, 3rd edn. Edinburgh: Churchill Livingstone.

Prady J, Vale A, Hill J (1998) Body image and sexuality. In: Hill J (ed) Rheumatology Nursing: a creative approach. Edinburgh: Churchill Livingstone, pp. 109-124.

Radojenic VP, Nicassio PM, Weisman MH (1992) Behaviour interventions with and without family support for rheumatoid arthritis. Behavioural Therapy 23: 13-30.

Rau R (2002) Adalimumab (a fully human anti-tumour necrosis factor alpha monoclonal antibody) in the treatment of active rheumatoid arthritis: the initial results of five trials. Annals of Rheumatic Diseases 61 Supp ii: 70-73.

Rawlins M, Chairman of NICE (2003) National Institute for Clinical Excellence (accessed online at www.nice.org.uk on 11 August).

Reid IR, Chapman GE, Fraser TRC et al (1986) Low serum osteocalcin levels in glucocorticosteroid-treated asthmatic. Journal of Clinical and Endocrinological Metabolism 62: 379-383.

Reif L (1975) Beyond medical intervention strategies for managing life in the face of chronic disease. In: Davis M, Kramer M, Straiss A (eds) Nurses in Practice. A perspective on work environments. St. Louis, MO: Mosby, pp. 261-273.

Reimsma R, Kirwan J, Taal E (2002) Patient education for adults with rheumatoid arthritis. The Cochrane Library. Oxford Software.

Rigby P, Glick EN, Smith R (1971) Intra-articular injection of triamcinolone in rheumatoid arthritis. MD Medicine Journal 19: 62-66.

Ritchlin C (2001) The role of cytokines in the spondyloarthropathies. Presentation at The emerging role of TNF inhibition in the treatment of spondyloarthropathies, American College of Rheumatology Meeting, San Francisco, CA.

Rizk TE, Pinals RS, Talaiver AS (1991) Corticosteroid injections in adhesive capsulitis: investigation of their value and site. Archives of Physical Medicine and Rehabilitation 72(1): 20-22.

Robinson DL, Anderson MM, Erpenbeck PM (1997) Telephone advice: new solutions for old problems. Nurse Practitioner 22: 179-192.

Robinson WH, Genovese MC, Moreland LW (2001) Demyelinating and neurologic events reported in association with tumour necrosis factor alpha antagonism. Arthritis and Rheumatism 44: 1977-1983.

Rodden C, Bell M (2002) Record keeping; developing good practice. Nursing Standard 17(1): 40-42.

Royal College of Nursing (1990) Unpublished survey of health authorities and their policies related to role extension for nurses. London: Royal College of Nursing.

Royal College of Nursing (1999) Nurse Telephone Consultation Services - information and good practice. London: Royal College of Nursing.

Royal College of Nursing (2000) Primary Care Trusts - a radical change in primary health care. London: Royal College of Nursing.

Royal College of Nursing (2001) Standards for Effective Practice and Audit in Rheumatology Nursing: guidance for nurses. London: Royal College of Nursing.

Royal College of Nursing (2002) A Charter for Rheumatology Nursing. London: Royal College of Nursing.

Royal College of Nursing (2003a) Guidance for Practitioners on the Assessment, Administration and Monitoring of Biologic Therapies for Inflammatory Arthritis. London: Royal College of Nursing.

Royal College of Nursing (2003b) Defining Nursing. London: Royal College of Nursing.

Ryan S (1996a) Defining the role of the specialist nurse. Nursing Standard 10(17): 27-29.

Ryan S (1996b) Living with rheumatoid arthritis; a phenomenological exploration. Nursing Standard 10(41): 45-48.

Ryan S (1997) Nurse led drug monitoring in the rheumatology clinic. Nursing Standard 11(24): 45-47.

Ryan S (1998) Psychological aspects. In: Hill J (ed.) Rheumatology Nursing: a creative approach. Edinburgh: Churchill Livingstone.

Ryan S, Dawes PT, Mayer B (1996) Does inflammatory arthritis affect sexuality? British Journal of Rheumatology 35(Supplement 2): 19.

Ryan S, Oliver S (2002) Rheumatoid arthritis. Nursing Standard 16(20): 45-52.

Ryan S, Hassell A, Dawes P, Kendall S (2003) Perceptions of control in patients with rheumatoid arthritis. Nursing Times 99(13): 36-38.

Scally G, Donaldson LJ (1998) Clinical governance and the drive for quality improvement in the new NHS in England. British Medical Journal 317: 61-65.

Schering Plough Ltd. (2003) Summary of Product Characteristics: infliximab. Hertfordshire: Schering Plough (accessed online at www.emc.vhn.net).

Schering Plough (2002) Summary of Product Characteristics: remicade. Hertfordshire: Schering Plough.

Scott DL, van Riel PL, van der Heijde D, Studnicka Benke A (1995) Assessing disease activity in rheumatoid arthritis. The Eular Handbook of Standard Methods. Sweden: Pharmacia.

Seedhouse D (2000) Practical Nursing Philosophy: the universal ethical code. Chichester: John Wiley & Sons.

Semple Piggot C (1996) Business Planning for NHS Management. London: Kogan Page.

Seradge H, Anderson MG (1990) Clostridial myonecrosis following intra-articular steroid injection. Clinical Orthopaedic Research 147: 207-209.

Shaul MP (1995) From early twinges to mastery; the process of adjustment in living with rheumatoid arthritis. Arthritis Care Research 8: 290-297.

Sheaff R (1996) The Need for Healthcare. London: Routledge.

Sieper J, Braun J, Rudwaleit M, Boonen A, Zink A (2002) Ankylosing spondylitis: an overivew. Annals of Rheumatic Diseases 61 Supp iii: 8-18.

Simon GE, VonKorff M, Rutter C, Wagner E (2000) Randomised trial of monitoring feedback and management of care by telephone to improve treatment of depression in primary care. British Medical Journal 320: 550-554.

Smart S (1994) Evaluating the impact: using a business planning approach. In: Humphris D (ed.) The Clinical Nurse Specialist. Houndswell: Macmillan, pp. 71-83.

Sparling M, Malleson P, Wood B, Petty R (1990) Radiographic follow up of joints injected with triamcinalone hexacetonide for the management of childhood arthritis. Arthritis and Rheumatism 33: 821-826.

Stark C, Christie P, Marr AC (1994) Running an emergency helpline. British Medical Journal 309: 44-45.

Stein MJ, Wallston KA, Nicassio PM (1988) Factor structure of the Arthritis Helplessness Index. Journal of Rheumatology 15: 427-432.

Stenger AA, Van Leeuwen MA, Houtman PM et al. (1998) Early effective suppression of inflammation in rheumatoid arthritis reduces radiographic progression. British Journal of Rheumatology 37: 1157-1163.

Strand V (2002) American College of Rheumatology Clinical Symposium: Drug toxicity. Conference proceedings (accessed online at www.rheumatology.org).

Stuart A, Rogers S, Modell M (2000) Evaluation of a direct doctor-patient telephone advice line in general practice. British Journal of General Practice 50: 305-306.

Sutcliffe AM (1999) A regional nurse led osteoporosis clinic. Nursing Standard 13(37): 46-47.

Swain RA, Kaplan B (1995) Practices and pitfalls of corticosteroid injection. The Physician and Sports Medicine 23(3): 27-40.

Symmons D, Bankhead C (1994) Health Care Needs Assessment for Musculoskeletal Diseases; the first step - estimating the number of incident and prevalent cases. Chesterfield: Arthritis Research Campaign.

Temmink D, Hutten JBF, Francke AL (2001) Rheumatology outpatient nurse clinics: a valuable edition? Arthritis Care Research 45: 280-286.

Thomson R, Lavender M, Madhok R (1995) How to ensure that guidelines are effective. British Medical Journal 311: 237-242.

Thwaites C, Carr M, Huggett A, Hughes RA (2000) Telephone helplines. Rheumatology 39: 78.

Thwaites C, Carr M, Hughes RA, Huggett A (2003) Patient preference for mode of delivery of telephone helpline:direct response versus answerphone. Rheumatology 42 Supp 1: 150.

Tijhuis GT, Zwinderman AH, Hazes JMW et al. (2002) A randomized comparison of care provided by a clinical nurse specialist, an inpatient team, and a day patient team in rheumatoid arthritis. Arthritis Care Research 47: 525-531.

Tingle J (1997) Pathways of care. In: Johnson S (ed.) Pathways of Care, Clinical Guidelines and the Law. Oxford: Blackwell, pp. 191-203.

Tingle J (2002) The professional standard of care in clinical negligence. British Journal of Nursing 11: 1375-1378.

Tremblay M, Dunn L (2002) Leading Leadership: navigating the leader's journey. National Nursing Practice Leadership Newsletter Autumn/Winter.

Tugwell P, Bombardier C (1982) A methodologic framework for developing and selecting endpoints in clinical trials. Journal of Rheumatology 9: 758-762.

Tugwell P, Bombardier C, Buchanan WW et al. (1990) Methotrexate in rheumatoid arthritis: impact on quality of life assessed by traditional standard item and individualized patient preference health status questionnaires. Archives of Internal Medicine 150: 59-62.

Tugwell P, Welch V, Suarez-Almazor M, Shea B, Wells G (2000) Efficacy and toxicity of old and new disase modifying antirheumatic drugs. Annals of Rheumatic Diseases 59 Supp I: 32-35.

Tunney AM (2003) Chart busters. Nursing Standard 17(36): 17-18.

Turesson C, Jacobsson L, Bergstrom U (1999) Extra-articular rheumatoid arthritis: prevalence and mortality. Rheumatology 38: 668-674.

Turnbull A (1987) Anaemia in rheumatoid arthritis, does it matter? Collected Reports on Rheumatic Disease. Chesterfield: Arthritis Research Campaign.

United Kingdom Central Council for Nursing, Midwifery and Health Visiting (1992) The Scope of Professional Practice. London: UKCC.

United Kingdom Central Council for Nursing, Midwifery and Health Visiting (1993) Final Report on the Future of Professional Practice. London: UKCC.

United Kingdom Central Council for Nursing, Midwifery and Health Visiting (2002) Report on the higher level of practice pilot and project. Executive Summary. London: UKCC.

van der Heijde D, Bird HA, Dougados M (1996) Baillière's Clinical Rheumatology. International Practice and Research 10(3): 43-45.

van der Heijde D, Braun J, McGonagle D, Siegel J (2002) Treatment trial in ankylosing spondylitis: current and future considerations. Annals of Rheumatic Diseases 61 Supp iii: 24-32.

van Leeuwen MA, van Rijswijk MH, van der Heijde DM et al. (1993) The acute-phase response in relation to radiographic progression in early rheumatoid arthritis: a prospective study during the first three years of the disease. British Journal of Rheumatology 32(Supplement 3): 9-13.

van Riel PLCM, Scott DL (2000) EULAR Handbook of Clinical Assessments in Rheumatoid Arthritis. The Netherlands: Zan Zuiden.

Verbrugge L (1985) Gender and health: an update on hypothesis and evidence. Journal of Health and Social Behaviour 26: 156-182.

Wahlberg AC, Cedersund E, Wredling R. (2003) Telephone nurses' experience of problems with telephone advice in Sweden. Journal of Clinical Nursing 12: 37-45.

Walsh M (2001) Nursing Frontiers. Accountability and the boundaries of care. Oxford: Butterworth Heinemann.

Ware J, Sherbourne C (1992) The MOS 36 item short form health survey (SF-36). Medical Care 30: 473-83.

Weinblatt M, Keystone EC, Furst DE et al. (2003) Adalimumab, a fully human anti-tumour necrosis factor alpha monoclonal antibody, for the treatment of rheumatoid arthritis in patients taking concomitant methotrexate. Arthritis and Rheumatism 48: 35-45.

Weitoft T, Uddenfeldt P (2000) Importance of synovial fluid aspiration when injecting intra-articular corticosteroids. Annals of Rheumatic Disease 59: 233-235.

White C (1998) Fatigue and sleep. In: Hill J (ed.) Rheumatology Nursing: a creative approach. Edinburgh: Churchill Livingstone, pp. 155-171.

White C (1998) Smooth Operator. Nursing Times 41: 44-45.

Willams P, Gumpel A (1990) Aspiration and injection of joints (1). British Medical Journal 281: 1990-1992.

Wilson Barnett J (1984) The Key Functions in Nursing: the fourth Winifred Raphael Memorial Lecture. London: Royal College of Nursing.

Wolfe F (1997) Adverse drug reaction of disease modifying anti-rheumatic drugs and DC-ARTs in rheumatoid arthritis. Clinical and Experimental Rheumatology 15 Supp 17: S75-S81.

Wolfe F, Zwillich SH (1998) The long-term outcomes of rheumatoid arthritis: a 23 year prospective, longitudinal study of total joint replacement and its predictors in 1,600 patients with rheumatoid arthritis. Arthritis and Rheumatism 41: 1072-1082.

World Health Organization (1983) The principles of quality assurance. Copenhagen: World Health Organization.

Wright S (1995) The role of the nurse: extended or expanded. Nursing Standard 9(33): 25-29.

Wyeth (2003) Summary of Product Characteristics: enbrel. Berkshire: Wyeth.

Yelin E, Callahan L (1995) The economic cost and social and psychological impact of musculoskeletal conditions. Arthritis and Rheumatism 38: 1351-62.

Zigmond AS, Snaith RP (1983) The Hospital Anxiety and Depression scale. Psychiatrica Scandinavica 67: 361-370.

Further reading

Adair J (1990) Understanding Motivation. London: Kogan Page.

Bathon JM, Martin RW, Fleischmann RM, Tesser JR, Schiff MH, Keystone EC, Genovese M, Wasko M, Moreland LW, Weaver AL, Markenson J, Fink BK (2000) A comparison of etanercept and methotrexate in patients with early rheumatoid arthritis. New England Journal of Medicine 343: 1586-1593.

Berne E (1970) Games People Play. Harmondsworth: Penguin.

Bernhard L, Walsh M (1995) Leadership - the key to professionalization of nursing. St Louis, MO: Mosby.

Byrne J (1998) Medication in rheumatic disease. In: Hill J (ed.) Rheumatology Nursing: a creative approach. Edinburgh: Churchill Livingstone

Carr AJ and Donovan JL (1998) Why doctors and patients disagree. British Journal of Rheumatology 37: 1-5.

Covey S (1993) 7 habits of highly effective people. London: Simon & Schuster.

Dieppe P, Doherty M, Macfarlane DG, Maddison P (1985) Rheumatological Medicine. Edinburgh: Churchill Livingstone.

Dimond B (2002) Legal Aspects of Nursing. Europe: Prentice Hall.

Ferrari R, Cash J, Maddison P (2000) Rheumatology Guidebook. Oxford: Bios Scientific Publishers.

Hill J (1998) Rheumatology Nursing: a creative approach. Edinburgh: Churchill Livingstone.

Hill J, Ryan S (2000) A Handbook for Community Nurses. London: Whurr.

Hunt G, Wainwright P (1994) Expanding the Role of the Nurse: the scope of professional practice. Oxford: Blackwell Science.

Kleinmann A (1988) The Illness Narrative: suffering healing and the human condition. New York: Harper Collins.

Long A, Scott DL (1997) Measuring Outcomes in Rheumatoid Arthritis. London: Royal College of Physicians.

McCann S, Weinman J (1996) Empowering the patient in the consultation: a pilot study. Patient Education and Counselling 27: 227-234.

Morrell C, Harvey G (2001) The Clinical Audit Handbook: improving the quality of health care. London: Baillière Tindall.

Peters T (1988) Thriving on Chaos. New York: Harper Collins

Rolfe G, Fulbook P (1999) Advanced Nursing Practice. Oxford: Butterworth-Heinemann.

Royal College of Nursing (1995) Telephone Helplines - guidelines for good practice. London: Telephone Helpline Group/Broadcasting Support Services, Royal College of Nursing.

Ryan S (1999) Drug Therapy in Rheumatology Nursing. London: Whurr.

Shekelle PG, Woolfe SH, Eccles M, Grimshaw J (1999) Developing guidelines. British Medical Journal 318: 593-596.

Woolf A, St John Dixon A (1998) Osteoporosis. A clinical guide. London: Martin Dunitz.

Index